CHINESE MASSAGE

Written by Bian Chunqiang and Tao Yu

Photographed by Jing Qiang and Ma Qianli

Translated by Hu Zhaoyun

Version revised by Harold Swindall

Shandong Friendship Press

First Edition 1996
ISBN—80551—828—9/R·12

Published by
Shandong Friendship Press
Shengli Street, Jinan, China
Printed by
Shandong Dezhou Xinhua Printing House
Distributed by
China International Book Trading Corporation
35 Chegongzhuang Xilu, Beijing 100044, China
P. O. Box 399, Beijing, China

Printed in the People's Republic of China

plumping the chest, treating facial paralysis, baldness and acne. Of course these disorders are not life-threatening. It aims at effecting a cure by gradually and fundamentally self-regulating the body. Of course it can be coordinated by appropriate media to achieve particular curative effects.

As to the locations to be beautified, beauty massage can be classified into the whole body and local parts. For the whole body, massage is performed all over the body. For local parts, massage may be performed along the meridians, on selected acupoints or on certain other locations. Usually it is performed on acupoints selected on certain locations, with the face as the major location. Massage may be performed on appropriate meridians and parts selected according to the aims of the beautification. In practice the selection of locations is interrelated, only the stresses are different.

As to the techniques of massage, the patterns of massage can be classified into dots, lines and planes; the speeds can be classified into rapid, unhurried and slow; the forces can be classified into heavy, moderate and light; the depths can be classified into shallow, moderate and deep; and the degrees of qi can be classified into strong, moderate and weak. In one word, the technique should be appropriate according one's own needs.

The Scope of Application and Contraindications of Beauty Massage

The mechanism of beauty massage determines its extensive scope of application.

For healthy people, beauty massage may help conserve and enhance the quality of health, resist aging, delay skin flaccidity, prevent the emergence of wrinkles and pigmented spots on the skin, strengthen skin resiliency, and make the skin fine, smooth and shiny. If born a beauty, one may still preserve the charms and graces as one's age increases.

The scope of application of beauty massage is as follows:

Pale, sallow or dim complexion, wrinkles, freckles, acne, chillblains, scars, smallpoxes, facial spasm and facial paralysis;

Dizziness, headache, trigeminal neuralgia, insomnia, baldness, myopia, hyperopia, strabismus, palpebral edema, blephraptosis, periophthalmic cyanosis, ophthalmic convulsion, rhinitis, brandy nose, tinnitus, deafness, toothache, agomphosis, gingival atrophy, ulcerative stomatitis, ozostomia, xerostomia and orolingual sores;

Pachylosis, muscular pain, cervical spondylosis, difficult activity of the joints, pathologic leanness, obesity, hypermastia, levelness of breast, mastoptosis and crater nipple.

Besides, beauty massage is also effective for internal and gynecological diseases slightly different from beautification in relationship. They will not be enumerated here.

Scope of contraindications. Heavy massage is contraindicated in cases of hunger, overeating, overfatigue and drunkenness, and during menstrual period, pregnancy and puerperium of females.

Massage is prohibited in the following cases:

Various kinds of acute and fulminating infectious diseases still in the infective period;

Ulceration, burn, scald, injury and chemical erosion of the skin at the locations to be beautified, and infectious dermatosis not yet cured;

Patients suffering from fracture, dislocation or hemorrhagic tendency at the locations to be beautified, or hemorrhagic diseases in bleeding period;

Congenital physiological deficiencies, and

hereditary diseases; various kinds of acute, dangerous and severe cases; tumor patients, and patients suffering from serious organic diseases;

Various kinds of mental diseases and psychoneuroses in the stage of attack; and those who will show serious adverse reactions after massage.

Points About the Attitude for Beauty Massage

The following are points of attitude for beauty massage.

Determination and cheefulness. Beauty massage is not merely the application of external force, but, more importantly, mental and physical exercise. The practice of beauty massage requires a good spiritual state. In a good spiritual state, the mind can be tranquilized, health can be built up, rapid effects can be achieved, and twice the result with half the effort can be got. Practice shows it is difficult for those with a poor spiritual state to get even half the result with twice the effort.

Confidence and perseverance. Beauty massage can achieve effects only through persevering exercise. Lack of perseverance will achieve little effect. The goals of longevity and pretty looks cannot be attained with a few instances of beauty massage, and beauty cannot be effected in a short time. "Constant efforts yield sure success"; practice with perseverance will in the course of time result in health, longevity and everlasting beauty.

Carefulness in assiduous exercise. With the mastery of the basic laws and techniques of beauty massage, it is also necessary to arrange exercise time scientifically. Exercise is prohibited immediately after meals, when hungry or when one needs to relieve himself. Exercise should be moderate during the menstrual period or pregnancy for females. The amount of exercise should be appropriate. Massage media should be used properly. Have a little rest after an exercise, and clean the body with warm water. Trim the fingernails properly, otherwise they will alter the effect of the exercise.

Avoid wind. This means beauty massage should be performed in a clean room with moderate temperature and avoid the invasion of wind. "Wind is the first pathogenic agent," so many diseases result from exposure to pathogenic wind. Old people, people suffering from chronic diseases and weak people must pay special attention to it. During exercise the pores are open, so pathogenic wind may cause serious diseases. The saying "Avoiding wind is like avoiding arrows" is really justified.

Avoid fatigue. This not only means that exercise is prohibited in case of extreme fatigue, but more importantly means that sexual activity should be moderate during the exercise period. Practice shows that after a period of exercise, especially the exercise of the method of reinforcing the essence, some people may achieve the reinforcement of *yang* and feel full of energy. At such time, sexual strain should particularly be avoided. Conservation and protection of essence and primordial *qi* will be beneficial to good health and beauty. Otherwise, intemperance in sexual life will spoil all the previous efforts, and beauty will be out of the question.

Coordination with sleep, diet, exercise and medical treatment.

With good rest, one will be energetic, vigorous and ready to do things. As for rest, sleep is the most important. People without sound sleep cannot be healthy, vigorous and beautiful. In the period of exercise, enough sleep must be guaranteed. Never eat and drink excessively. Beauty massage can be coordinated with walking, trotting, shadow boxing and other dynamic exercises. It should be well coordinated with medical treatment. Diseases should be treated in time lest the chances of cure be missed and the illness aggravated. It is important to combine exercise and proper care. "It is lost labor to exercise without proper care" is a good piece of advice.

The techniques of beauty massage and the movements of exercises should be as accurate as possible, and be applied freely and correctly. Autonomy, naturalness and smoothness are advocated to better activate the potentials of the body, achieve self-controlled disease-preventing and anti-aging effects and bring about eternal beauty.

The Media and Instruments of Beauty Massage

Determined by the locations and aims of beauty massage, besides bare-hand performance on oneself or others, sometimes certain instruments are needed to help carry out the performance, In addition, to achieve skin beauty effects such as smoothness, fairness, delicacy, fineness and prettiness, massage media such as oil, ointment, cream, liquors and juices of various forms are usually used. Sometimes this is coordinated with baths in medicated or other necessary solutions.

Common Media

Massage media can not only protect the skin, but can also take advantage of the force and other information of massage and perform their permeating, nourishing and medical functions to enhance the beautifying effects. For those with beautification obstacles, such as pachylosis, freckles or latent sores, the selection of media should vary according to necessity and conditions. One should not follow suit blindly and apply creams, for example, at random. Otherwise, the consequences will be dreadful. The forms and types of beauty massage media are diversified, and most have a medical effect. The forms can be classified into juice, water, oil, vinegar, wine, honey, ointment, decoction, powder, cream, and pills. The media can be fruits, pollens, egg, milk or drugs. These can be self-prepared, cheap and convenient.

The application of beauty massage media can be roughly divided into three cases: massage followed by smearing, massage and smearing at the same time and smearing followed by massage.

Fruits commonly used are as follows:

Banana, rich in vitamins, especially effective for dry and sensitive skin;

Papaya, suitable for neutral or dry skin;

Lemonade, suitable for oilly skin;

Walnut kernel oil, having nourishing effect on dry and allergic skin;

Pineapple, able to make the skin fine and smooth;

Tomato, cucumber, watermelon, white gourd, Chinese yam, potato and carrot all contain large amounts of vitamins and trace elements. They can be eaten as food, their pulp can be applied to the face, or their juice can be smeared on the face, all to be coordinated with slight massage.

Fruits such as apple, pear, orange, longan and beet contain rich sugar, tannin and vitamins. As convenient beauty media common to all families, they can be selected according to necessity.

Egg white and milk can tighten the skin, eliminate coarse skin and filth and whiten the skin, and is suitable for skin of various kinds. Sour milk, salad oil, butter milk and fresh milk are slightly astringent and can make the skin clean, fine, smooth and shiny.

Media prepared with common medicinal herbs can be used to treat or prevent various dermatoses affecting beauty. For example, safflower-chicken oil ointment can treat chapped skin; ginger slices can be used to scrub the scalp to treat baldness; trichosanthes soap can remove filth and shine the skin; flavescent sophora liquor can treat the itching of dry and moist skin; chrysanthemum or peppermint water can moisten and freshen the skin; Chinese ilex oil can treat rubella and stop itching; menthocamphorate can treat insect bites; and Chinese angelica and safflower preparation can moisten the skin and beautify the face. Traditional Chinese medicines have plentiful and extensive therapeutic effects, and usually have no adverse effects. There are broad prospects for their exploitation. It can be safely said that the best future natural beauty media are bound to emerge from traditional Chinese medicines.

As for the media commonly seen in the market, such as vaseline, massage oil, apricot kernel oil, malt oil, rose oil, olive oil, spot-removing oil and skin-moistening cream, they should be selected carefully and should not be abused.

Here it should be particularly pointed out that, as recorded in ancient Chinese books and as proved by modern practice, saliva can treat acne: after bare — hand beauty massage of the face, wash the hands, dip in the saliva produced by stirring the tongue in the mouth and smear the saliva on the face. Studies show that saliva contains many kinds of enzymes and germicidal and sterilizing elements and has digestive and immunological functions. Thus, this self-produced precious and convenient medium might be tried.

Besides, at home one may select appropriate dressing to make a face membrane which is both economical and practical. There are many ways to make face membranes, and many kinds of membrane to be made. The following are a few easy ways.

Appropriate amount of fresh egg, honey, skimmed milk powder and fine flower, add appropriate amount of boiled water, mix them well into a paste, and spread it on the face, the neck or the back of the hands, When it is dry (after about 40 minutes), rinse it off with warm water. On cold days, the paste may be slightly heated and then applied. Such a mask can increase skin nourishment and make the skin clean and fine. It can be used at home in all seasons.

Slice various fruits such as cucumber, white gourd, watermelon, tomato, orange and citrus and spread the slices on the face, or pound the fruits into a paste and apply it on the face. Half and hour later, wipe the face with a soft warm towel. This method can whiten the skin, diminish the pores and make the skin fine and delicate.

Prepare 1 part of honey, 1/2 part of glycerine, 1 gram of VC tablet, 3 parts of water and 1 part of fine flour, mix them into a paste and apply it to the face. Half an hour later, rinse it off with clear water. This method can make the skin fine and smooth.

Prepare 5 parts of white vinegar and 1 part of glycerin, mix them well, then add appropriate amount of clean and very fine talcum power, mix them into a paste and apply it. This method can make rough skin fine and delicate.

Soak 30 grams of trichosanthes in hot water. Add appropriate Chinese yam powder, mix them into a paste and apply it to the face. This method can effectively remove spots and latent sores, and can moisten and whiten the skin as well.

The above-mentioned are a few simple methods. Many face membranes are sold in market, including nourishing ones such as ginseng, pearl and vitamin face membranes and medical ones such as anti-comedo face membrane, stain-removing face membrane and whitening face membrane. They are of different grades and may be selected according to different needs.

Many beauty media can be coordinated with bathing, and this is bathing beautification. To clean and moisten the skin of the whole body is the aim of bathing, and an important indispensable link of beautification as well.

Besides plain-water bathing, bathing beautification also resorts to medicinal bathing, examples of which are introduced in the following:

Chrysanthum-honey bathing: Dry chrysanthemum 40 grams and honey 15 grams. First boil the chrysanthum in a pot gently for 20 minutes, remove the residue and pour the extract into the bath water, then add the honey, mix them well, and have a bath in it. Long-term bathing can remove wrinkles, and make the skin shiny, clean and fine; it can also make one spirited and impressive.

Trichosanthes-lotus-vinegar bathing: Chinese trichosanthes 30 grams, lotus leaf 20 grams (fresh leaf 40 grams), and vinegar 5 grams. Add water and boil them for 30 minutes. Remove the residue and add the extract into the bath water, then add the vinegar, and have a bath in it. This method can treat skin driness and rubella, and can remove wrinkles, stop itching, and soften and moisten the skin.

Schizonepeta-ledebouriella-dahurian angelica-defatted milk powder bathing: Schizonepeta spike 10 grams, ledebouriella 10 grams, dahurian angelica 10 grams and defatted milk powder 20 grams. Boil the three medicinal herbs for 20 minutes. Then mix the milk powder into the extract and add them into the bath water, and have a bath in it. This method has good effects on allergic skin and for those liable to suffer from eruption of smallpoxes.

Flavescent sophora-cnidium bathing: Flavescent sophora 20 grams, cnidium fruit 20 grams and peppermint 10 grams. Add water and boil them. Remove the residue and add the extract into the bath water and have a bath in it. This method is applicable to females with skin suceptible to infection and pruritus genitalium.

Five-flower bathing: Chrysanthemum 10 grams, honeysuckle flower 10 grams, safflower 10 grams, Chinese rose 10 grams, and rose 10 grams. Soak them for an hour and boil them gently for 10 minutes. Press the residue and add the extract into the bath water, and have a bath in it. This method can make the skin fine, delicate, moist, smooth and fragrant. This method can prevent and treat papular allergy of the skin.

Besides the above-mentioned medicinal bathings, there are also food bathings, for example, oatmeal bathing, milk, honey plus fruit juice bathing, and rose oil bathing. Some of them are very expensive, with complicated processes, so they will not be introduced in detail here.

It is to be pointed out that, when bathing

with plain water, one may, according to the rules of beauty massage introduced later, rub, scrub or knead the body from the lower part to the upper part and from the inner side to the outer side with a sponge, a towel or bare hands, conducting massage while bathing. This will be very beneficial. But note that the water temperature cannot be too high, otherwise, long-term bathing will make the skin flaccid.

Common Instruments

Massage instruments are only convenient accessories. In cases of weak physique or locations unreachable for the hands during self-massage, appropriate instruments may be employed.

Any object, as long as it is not harmful and is convenient and able to produce good effects, can be selected as a massage instrument. Instruments suitable to one's own conditions can be selfmade according to one's needs.

The instruments vary with the locations to be massaged. Instruments for acupoints are round-headed or pointed, such as rubber mallets and wood awls (a kind of massage rod). Instruments for meridian lines include rings, slabs, ancient coins, cups, spoons, mugs, saucers, plates and bowls made of jade, horn, porcelain or metal. Those whose edges are delicate, hard, smooth and moist are the best ones. They can be wetted with water and be used to scrape or scrub certain meridian lines, thus properly stimulating the skin and achieving certain beautifying effects. Instruments for the whole face include wood combs, towels, bath towels, brushes, mulberry rods and rods made of bamboo or rattan , as well as instrumerts with specific shapes (finger, palm, fist or ball) made of rubber, plastic or other materials. Some of them can be used to punch or press, some to scrape along the meridians, and some to percuss certain locations.

In addition, along with the development of science and technology, various electric massage devices, massage mattresses and massage chairs as well as weight-loss massage devices and breast-plumping massage devices made for special purposes have also entered the market.

It must be pointed out that such instruments are not human beings; mechanical force cannot replace the force, qi, energy and effect of human massage, and dependence on instrument cannot attain the goal of beautification. Instruments are only accessories. To achieve real and everlasting beautiful looks and a healthy body, one must rely on one's own hands and willpower.

Part II

The Functional Mechanism of Beauty Massage

The Functional Mechanism of Beauty Massage

Chinese beauty massage employs unique health-building and beautifying means with traditional Chinese medical characteristics, activates and initiates the health-building and beautifying potentials of the human body, effects health and longevity and yields natural beauty. Numerous facts show that long-term correct massage can definitely preserve health, prolong life, prevent diseases and produce beauty. Drugs, however good, cannot match its beauty. It is this charm that attracts people to explore its mysteries. Its practice and studies prove that its mechanism is very complicated, whether viewed from the theories of both traditional Chinese and Western medicine, or from the achievements of many modern scientific researches. The following is a brief exploration from these three views.

View from traditional Chinese medicine

A. Balancing *yin* and *yang* and regulating the *Zang-Fu* organs (the viscera). The *ying-yang* and five-element theories are the basic theories of traditional Chinese medicine and the basis of the diagnosis and treatment according to overall analysis of symptoms and signs. The *zang-fu*, *ying-wei* and *qi*-blood theories are important components of the theories of traditional Chinese medicine. "Imbalance of *yin* and *yang*" is the fundamental reason for diseases. The Chapter "Grand Discussion on the Concept of *Yin* and *Yang* Reflected by Various Natural and Life Phenomena" in *Plain Questions* says: "*Yin* and *yang* are the doctrines of the universe, the principles of all things, the parents of changes, the province of life and death, and the home of wonder. Treatment of diseases must be directed against their roots." The five-element theory deals with the promoting, restraining, encroaching and counterrestraining relations among the five natural substances of Wood, Fire, Earth, Metal and Water. It is an age-old philosophic thought and a theory used to analyze, study, explain and predict the relations and laws of the changes of things.

When it is applied to traditional Chinese medicine, the five elements are associated with the liver, heart, spleen, lung and kidney respectively; the theory deals with the physiological and pathological relations such as exterior and interior, deficiency and excess and cold and heat among the *Zang-Fu* organs; and this forms the viscera-state doctrine. Appropriate massage may balance *yin* and *yang* and regulate the viscera. "*Yin* and *yang* in equilibrium" will lead to good health; the result of imbalance will be morbidity. Haggard complexion, dim skin, acne and macular eruption are manifestations of discord of the viscera and imbalance to *yin* and *yang*. Massage is beneficial to the viscera, so it can surely effect beauty.

B. Reinforcing the fundamentals, eliminating the pathogenic factors and regulating *qi* and blood. "The sun, the moon and the stars are the three treasures of heaven, and essence, *qi* and vitality are the three treasures of man." Essence is the root of life, *qi* is the source of energy and vitality is the basis of man. These are the basic elements that maintain the life of a person. *Qi* and blood are the foundation of these elements. If *qi* and blood are sufficient, one will be healthy; if *qi* and blood are deficient, one will be weak; if *qi* and blood are impeded, one will be ill; and if qi and blood are stagnant, one will die. The life activities of a person rely on nutritious and defensive qi and blood for nourishment and maintenance. The health and beauty of human skin is directly related to the changes of qi and blood. Rough skin, dim complexion, acne and macular eruption are related to the derangement of qi and blood, either stagnancy of qi and stasis of blood or disharmony between nutritious and defensive qi and blood. Massage promotes   ind blood, "tonifying the deficie   the excessive." Practice shows th   hes doing a set of beauty massage,   feel more energetic and refresh   of time beauty will be inevitabl   gevity and vigorousness will be

C. Dredging the meridians and lubricating the joints. The meridians are the channels in which human qi and blood flow. They connect with the skin outwardly and with the viscera inwardly, sending the nutritrients of foodstuff to the entire body, moistening the skin, replenishing the striae of skin, strengthening muscles and bones, nourishing the viscera, managing the opening and closing, and resisting the invasion of pathogenic factors. It is these meridians that "reflect outwardly what is inward", reflecting in the health and beauty or weakness and ugliness of the facial skin whether the *qi* and blood of the viscera are sufficient or insufficient, good or bad, and whether their circulation is normal or not. However, benigh therapeutic information may through massage stimulate the acupoints of the body, produce energy and enable *qi* and blood to circulate over the entire body along the widespread meridians, thus influencing the viscera and other parts. So massage on the surface of the body may treat the disorders of the interior organs, and massaging specific acupoints may produce beautifying effects—owing to the connecting functions of the meridians. Chinese beauty massage by no means presses whatever is not beautiful, nor treats the head for a headache or the foot for a footache, exerting force mechanically. Instead it is a set of rigorous, dialectical and flexible methods based on the concept of the whole. For example, massage for baldness is not performed merely on the head, but also on some acupoints under the knees and on the soles along certain meridian lines. Of course this must be based on the differentiation of symptoms and signs, and can be practiced after a sure diagnosis. This is a characteristic of traditional Chinese medicine. It is also under the guidance of this dialectical thought that beauty massage has incessantly summarized the precious experience of the forerunners, found the general laws, understood the special phenomena and formed a regular and relatively complete set of medical skills.

Viewed from the theories of modern medicine:

A. Benign massage, as a physical stimulating agent, through nervous segmental reflection and the reflection, diffusion and feedback of the interior organs of the body, causes a series of responsive reflection and directly or through the nervous system acts on the incretory organs to regulate the nerves, humors of the body and the functions of the incretory organs to a finer level. For example, when the cerebral cortex is under benign protective stimulation, the coordination of the domains of the brain may be synchronized and ordered, and the endocrines may be properly coordinated, thus improving the blood circulation and the nourishment of the various systems of organs and regulating them to a fine physiological state. When one is healthy, one is beautiful naturally.

B. Through the reflection of the nervous system, massage can promote the tissues to release active histamine and acetylcholine, further strengthening blood circulation; promote metabolism; produce a series of physiological, functional and informational recovery beneficial to the normal life, health and beauty of the organism; invigorate the beneficial factors of the respiratory, digestive, motory, nervous, urinary, reproductive and incretory systems; and exert a marked influence on the health and beauty of the body.

C. Massage can not only exert influence on blood dynamics and cause temporary blood redistribution, but can also increase the amount of red blood cells, white blood cells, blood platelets and hemoglobins in the blood; strengthen the bacteriophagocytic power of white blood cells and serum alexic titer; it can also strengthen the irritable reaction of the hypothysis-adrenocortical system and sympathoadrenal medullary system and the protective system of the body against various harmful stimulations and strengthen its immunity. The strengthening of the internal vitality will effect the health and beauty of the human body.

D. The psychological and physical delight and

enjoyment beauty massage brings may help get rid of worries and vexations. With concentration of spirit and cheerfulness of mind, marked effects can be produced. Practice shows that a fine state of psychology may greatly influence and promote the state of health and inevitably bring about fine looks.

E. Beauty massage acts on the skin, and can eliminate decrepit epidermal keratinocytes, improve cutaneous respiration, and increase the secretion of the sebaceous and sudoriferous glands, thus increasing the luster of the skin; the strengthening of the functions of the intradermal elastic fibers may increase the elasticity of the skin, thus increasing the protective action of the skin, benefiting the regulation of the body temperature; and building health and beautifying the skin.

F. Beauty massage has a great influence on the muscles. It can accelerate the elimination of the fatigue of tired muscles, enhance myodynamia, and improve the blood circulation in the muscles. Practice tells us that long-term persevering massage has marked effects on some myoatrophy patients. Massage may help those who lack beauty owing to pathogenic leanness gradually plump up and become smooth-skinned, muscular and beautiful.

Viewed from the achievements of some modern studies:

A. Massage from the viewpoint of information theory: Modern biological studies have revealed that the organs of the human body have specific biological information respectively (each has its own innate biological electricity or frequency). When a certain organ has a disorder, its relevant biological information will modify accordingly. Such information modification will affect the balance of the entire life system. Beauty massage, in the light of the viscera and meridian theories, acts on certain acupoints, and such benign stimulation will produce certain biological information which through the transmission system is transmitted into the organ concerned. As a result, the abnormal biological information will be regulated, the affected dynamic balance will change for the better, and health and beauty will be achieved.

B. From the viewpoint of cybernetics: At present, scientists hold that from the angle of cybernetics a human body can be regarded as a complete self-regulating control system. The brain is the center of this control system. Its task is to analyze and process the various kinds of information coming from both inside and outside the body. In normal conditions, the regulating and control system is in coordination to maintain life and preserve a state of health. In case of morbidity, the regulation and control will be "out of order". This needs to be "recuperated", and massage is one of the means of recuperation. Fine face beauty massage may change the out-of-order state of the center, rehabilitate the cerebral cortex and the entire body, recover its control function and facilitate the balance system in charge of autonomously regulating the life, health and beauty of the body to change toward a fine, new and effective dynamic balance.

C. From the viewpoint of the systems theory: The dysfunction of any system of the human body is without exception due to changes of its internal energy, and the disorder in one system will inevitably affect other systems. Effective regulation of the system suffering from changes of internal energy will recover the system to normality, eliminate the "crisis" of other systems at the same time and bring about the coordinated and ordered operations of all the systems. For example, for one with stagnancy of *qi* and stasis of blood, drug treatment coordinated with correct massage may cause changes of the internal energy of the qi and blood system, promote the flow of qi and blood circulation, eliminate the disorder of stagnancy of qi and stasis of blood, and produce the beauty effect of "rosy complexion".

D. From the viewpoint of the steady-state theory: The theory of self-control steady-state regulation related to the body and mind, which has been applied by traditional Chinese medicine for thousands of years, has been gaining increasing attention of many countries recently, and has become an advanced branch of life science. One of the basic principles of Chinese beauty massage is the "integration of form and mentality", "integration of body and mind" or "integration of activity and inertia". This principle is identical with the viewpoint of modern medicine of body and mind.

E. From the viewpoint of microcirculation: Microcirculation scholars hold that the sound microcirculation function of an organism is the prerequisite to guarantee its normal physiological, functional and vital information and health and beauty information. When obstacles emerge in the microcirculation system, many diseases will occur, and health and beauty will be harmed. Massage is one of the most effective ways to recuperate microcirculation. For example, massage may warm the face and the palm, raise the local skin temperature, strengthen the local blood circulation, and surely produce beauty effects.

F. From the viewpoint of the mechanism of senility: Though factors influencing senility are many, including spiritual, physiological, environmental and social ones, study of its mechanism discloses that senility starts from cells, especially brain nervous cells, and the senility of cells occurs with the dysfunction of metabolism. Practice shows that for people in the same environmental conditions, those who can do self-care massage and do it perseveringly are definitely more healthy and beautiful than those who never do it. In recent years I have been teaching this massage to the students of a geriatric university. The statistics show that its results are convincing; that is, it delays the progress of senility and is beneficial to health, beauty and longevity.

G. From the viewpoint of holographism: Presently the latest theory, it derives from ancient Chinese philosophy— *The Book of Changes*. Holographism organically incorporates the visceral phenomena, meridians and *qi* and blood of traditional Chinese medicine, the theories of *qigong*, the doctrine of five elements' motion and six kinds of natural factors and the theory of time and space, and is practically applied to acupuncture and massage.

In short, along with the development of science, the precious legacy of traditional Chinese medicine has increasingly attracted the attention of the world. A complete theory of traditional Chinese medicine will be combined with modern medical science. The great theory and practice of combined Western and Chinese medicines will constantly reveal the mysteries of the mechanism of beauty massage. A beauty massage full of the characteristics of traditional Chinese medicine will surely be recognized and valued, and it will add grace to the beautification researches of the world.

The Viscera Theory and Beauty-Health Massage

The viscera theory of traditional Chinese medicine is the core of its theoretical system, and is an important theoretical foundation guiding its medical practice. Chinese beauty massage is also influenced by the theory.

The word "viscera" is a general term for the interior organs, including the five solid organs, the six hollow organs and extraordinary *fu*-organs. (It is to be noted that the viscera here are not anatomical entities and are classified according to their functions.) This chapter emphatically discusses the relation between the five solid organs and beautification. The five solid organs refer to the heart, the liver, the spleen, the lung and the kidney. *The Canon of Internal Medicine* says, "Internal states will be reflected outwardly." This means whether the functions of the five organs are normal or not will be directly reflected in the glow or gloom of the face. Thus, the skin of the face is referred to by some as "a mirror of the five organs".

The relationship between the viscera and beautification according to traditional Chinese medicine is as follows.

The heart and beautification

Located in the chest, the heart is the controller of mental activities and the headquarters of the meridians, and dominates life activities. The heart governs blood vessels and promotes blood circulation, making the organism nourished. Through the transmission of the meridians, the qi and blood from the heart flow upward to the face and the five sense organs. Only vigorous heart-qi and replete vessels can make a ruddy and lustrous complexion, dark hair and beard and shining eyes. This is why traditional Chinese medicine says "The complexion reflects the condition of the heart". That the heart governs mental activities means the heart decides the outward manifestations of the life activities of the human body, such as complexion, eye expression, posture, stature and temperament. If a person is spirited and vigorous, it means he or she has reached a higher realm of beautification.

The liver and beautification

Located in the abdominal cavity, the liver governs the flow of qi and is in charge of meditation. It regulates the flow of qi, determines the mood, dredges the bile and promotes the digestion and transmission of the spleen and kidney. The liver also stores blood. When blood is sufficient, the complexion will be ruddy; if liver-blood is insufficient, the complexion will be livid and dark. The liver has its specific body opening in the eye, and is in charge of the tendons. The fingernails reflect the condition of the liver. The normal physiological function of the liver is closely related to the brightness of the eyes, the luster of the fingernails and the robustness of the tendons.

The spleen and beautification

Located in the abdominal cavity, the spleen and stomach are "the basis of the acquired constitution". The function of the spleen and stomach is to digest food, transport nutrients, and keep qi, blood and body fluid flowing in vessels and meridians, thus maintaining life and nourishing the skin. The function of the spleen also includes transporting and transforming water-dampness. In case of hypofunction of the spleen, there will be water retention which may result in skin swelling and facial edema. If water dampness in long retention turns to heat, it will steam the face and cause acne and brandy nose. The spleen is in charge of sending up essential substances and refined nutritious substances and keeping the face sufficiently nourished. The mouth is the window of the spleen, and the spleen has its outward manifestation on the lips. If the spleen is sufficient with *qi* and blood the lips will be moist and ruddy. On the contrary, if the spleen is deficient with *qi* and blood, the lips will be dull-colored and short of luster.

The lung and beautification

Located in the thoracic cavity, the lung governs respiration. If respiration is impeded, how can the beauty of the skin be spoken of? The lung governs the defensive *qi* in the *qi* of the body. If the defensive *qi* is exuberant, the skin will be moist, lustrous, soft and beautiful, and the part between the skin and the flesh will be tight, enabling the skin to adapt to the changes of the weather and prevent the invasion of external pathogens. The dispersing function of the lung can distribute the food essence and body liquid transported by the spleen over the facial skin and make it soft and beautiful. The lung also has the function of dredging and regulating the water channels. It can maintain the normal flow and discharge of water, thus avoiding some disorders of the skin such as edema or shrivelling. All vessels converge in the lung, so it can help the flow of blood and improve facial blood circulation.

The kidney and beautification

Located on both sides of the lumbar vertebrae, the kidneys store essence and govern water, the reception of air, reproduction and growth. The kidney is the origin of congenital constitution. Kidney essence transforms into kidney-qi which keeps the functions of the five organs normal and makes qi and blood exuberant. Whether a person can enjoy longevity and fine complexion relies on the sufficiency of kidney-qi. If kidney-qi is insufficient, the face will have black spots. If the function of the kidney to govern water is disturbed, it will be incapable of proper regulation, and disorders such as limb edema and skin dryness will occur. The kidney dominates the bones and forms marrow; furthermore, "the teeth are the terminals of the bones", so the firmness and whiteness of the teeth also manifest the exuberance of kidney-qi. The hair manifests the condition of the kidney, so whether the hair is beautiful or not is closely related to it. If the kidney essence is insufficient, one will be old before one's time, with the hair becoming white or dry or falling before its time.

The Skin and Beauty-Health Massage

Since massage acts mainly on the skin, its first objective is to make the skin healthy and beautiful. For beauty massage especially, knowing the skin's structure is of primary importance.

Skin is the surface of the human body, and is the body's first line of defense, so it has the title of bodyguard. From its weight and area, the skin is the largest organ of the body. Its total weight makes up 16% of the weight of the body, and the area of the skin of an adult is about 1.5-2 square meters. Whether a person is healthy and beautiful or not can be reflected in the skin, so the skin is also a window and mirror of the human body.

On the surface of the skin there are many dermal ridges, dermal sulci and rugae which, under a high-power microscope, show a criss-cross network of ravines of different depths. On the dermal ridges there can be seen many small concave holes called pores, which are the openings of sweat ducts. Dermal sulci are formed by the arrangement and traction of the fibrous bundles in the skin tissues. Dermal sulci divide the dermal surface into many triangles, rhombuses and polygons, which are most clear in areas such as the back of the hand and the neck. Accumulation of skin excreta, skin secreta and outside dirt on the dermal sulci may affect the functions of the skin and even cause the aging of the skin, so it is very important to frequently clean the skin and keep it healthy.

The colors of the skin vary among individuals, and are closely related to factors such as race, age, sex and outside environment. Even for the same person, the colors of the skin at different locations are of different shades. The Chinese people belong to the yellow race, the pigments of their skin are relatively light. The skin of the young females especially is relatively thin, with well-developed subcutaneous tissues and plentiful dermal vessels, and is mostly fair and rosy.

The structure of the skin can be divided into three layers: the outer layer is the epiderm, the middle layer is the true skin, and the inner layer is the subcutaneous tissue. In the epiderm from the innermost layer to the outermost layer cells are constantly germinating and growing upward (called keratinization medically) until they exfoliate. The innermost layer is called the basal layer or the germinal layer, which is closely connected with the true skin and is formed by a layer of cylindrical cells. The basal layer cells keep dividing to make up for the exfoliated cells of the surface horny layer and repair the deficiencies of the epiderm. The outermost layer of the skin is the horny layer, composed by several layers of keratinized anuclear platycytes. Such cells are decrepit, and usually exfoliate to form scales. This layer can resist the light stimulation of acid and alkaline and prevent the invasion of water or bacteria.

The true skin is located under the epiderm, and is mainly composed of connective tissues (including collagenous fibers, elastic fibers, matrixes and cell components). Besides, it also has hair cortex, muscular tissues (erect hair muscles), capillaries, lymphatic vessels, nerves, sweat glands, sebaceous glands and sensory peripheral organs. The true skin has no power of regeneration, so its injuries will leave scars.

The subcutaneous tissue is the deepest layer of the skin, and is composed of a large amount of adipose tissues scattered among loose connective tissues. The latest researches show that the subcutaneous tissue can buffer outward impact, keep the body temperature, provide energy, and also promote the development of females and participate in the regulatory process of the maturity of female sexual glands. The skin also has many accessory organs, such as hair, hair follicles, sweat glands, sebaceous glands, fingernails and toenails.

The skin is the primary focus of beauty massage, and the skin of the face in particular occupies a decisive position in the beauty culture. Directly contacting the surface of the skin, beauty massage can eliminate the decrepit cells of the skin, regulate body temperature, strengthen sensory conduction, and increase the luster and elasticity of the skin. Massage can promote the dilation of capillaries, improve skin nourishment, and promote the circulation of blood and lymph. In recent years, some experimental data of massage show that massage can cause the decrepit cells of the skin epiderm to exfoliate and improve cutaneous respiration, to the benefit of the secretion of the glands. Forceful massage may cause the skin to produce a kind of substance called histamine which can activate the blood vessels and nerves of the skin to bring about capillarectasis and increase the speed and volume of blood flow, thus changing the color; it can also recover the elasticity for pale and sallow skin deficient of elasticity and enhancing its resistance against temperature and mechanical stimulations. So beauty massage has certain curative effects on rough skin, dark, lusterless, sallow and pale complexions, facial wrinkles and acne, promoting both the health and rosiness of the skin and curing the hidden factors that hamper skin beauty. Additionally massage can soften scars.

Wrinkling is a phenomenon of skin aging. Its causes include digestive dysfunction, long-term tension of the nerves, excessive anxiety, lowering of the hormone level, and impeded circulation of capillary blood and disturbance of the transportation of nutritious substances. Freckles are black or brown pigmented spots. Their appearance may be related to hereditary factors, weakening of hepatorenal functions or the increase of unusual pigmentary substances in the body. Among freckles, butterfly freckles are commonly seen during the menstrual period, gestational period and puerperium of females, with clear outlines and mostly symmetrical. Massage can regulate local blood supply, improve hepatorenal functions, balance the level of hormone secretion, promote blood circulation and remove blood stasis, and relieve inflammation and remove toxins, to attain the goal of eliminating wrinkles and removing freckles.

Beautiful and elegant hair may make one glow with vigor and grace. To protect and beautify your hair is an important element of the beauty culture. The hair is a kind of hairy substance with the longest hair shaft growing on the surface of the human body, with a very strong growth ability. According to studies of experts, the hair of a person in adolescence grows most vigorously, with about several hundred of hairs growing out each day. However, along with the increase of one's age, hypofunction of the body, especially deficiency of the kidney-essence, insufficiency of the liver blood and spleen-qi, or improper protection and nourishment may affect the growth and regeneration of the hair. There may occur early graying of the hair, baldness and even pelade, which all seriously affect beauty. The causes of baldness are many; however, no matter what kind of baldness, in most cases massage can, in coordination with other treatments, act on the central nervous system, improve nervous dysfunction, remove local vasospasm, promote the blood circulation and strengthen the nutrition intake of the hair and prevent or treat baldness.

Beauty Massage and Knowledge of Meridians and Acupoints

The theory of meridians (the theory of energetical channels and collaterals) is one of the bases of traditional Chinese medical theory. It runs through the physiology, pathology, diagnosis, treatment, beautology, health-care and other aspects of traditional Chinese medicine.

According to traditional Chinese medicine, the human body is composed of the five *Zang* organs and six *Fu* organs (the interior organs), the limbs, the five sensory organs, the skin, the hair and other tissues in combination. They have their respective unique physiological functions. They can well coordinate with each other and together maintain the normal operation of the whole organism precisely because the meridians have them closely connected. Owing to the distribution of the meridians, the interior and exterior and the left and right of the human body are closely linked to form a unified, dynamic and organic whole.

Through massage of specific meridians and acupoints, acupoint beauty masssage makes the skin lustrous, moist, healthy and beautiful while effectively preventing and treating many disorders affecting the looks to achieve beauty. Acupoint beauty massage has not only plentiful and scientific methods but also has a complete theoretical system, and is an important component of the series of beauty massage; furthermore, it is a beauty remedy with Chinese national characteristics. The methods of acupoint beauty massage are convenient, economical, safe and reliable. Besides, it combines prevention and treatment and incorporates health and beauty. Anybody, whether male or female, old or young, diseased or undiseased, strong or weak, fat or thin, as long as he or she knows the meridians and acupoints, understands the techniques and can perform them properly, can achieve the effects of health building and beautification.

Massaging the skin along the meridian lines is a traditional Chinese beauty method. In general practice the meridians commonly used are fourteen meridians, namely the Twelve Regular meridians plus the Conception Vessel and the Governor Vessel. In massage the meridians commonly used are the Twelve Regular Meridians and the Eight Extra Meridians. Among the Twelve Regular Meridians, the *Yin* meridians are *Zang* meridians, located on the inner sides of the trunk and limbs, and the *Yang* meridians are *Fu* organs, located on the outer sides of the trunk and limbs. Meridians distributed in the upper part of the body are termed Hand meridians, and those distributed in the lower part of the body are termed Foot meridians. The inner and outer sides of the trunk and limbs are divided into the front, middle and back parts, so there are three *Yin* meridians and three *Yang* meridians. The Conception Vessel is the meridian running along the front midline down across the neck, the chest and the belly, which controlls all the *Yin* meridians of the body. The Governor Vessel is the meridian running along the back midline up across the head, nape of the neck, back and waist, governing all the *Yang* meridians of the body.

For the convenience of memory, the circulation law of the Twelve Meridians can be summarized into one sentence: "Raise the hands and stand upright, then *Yin* ascends and *Yang* descends."

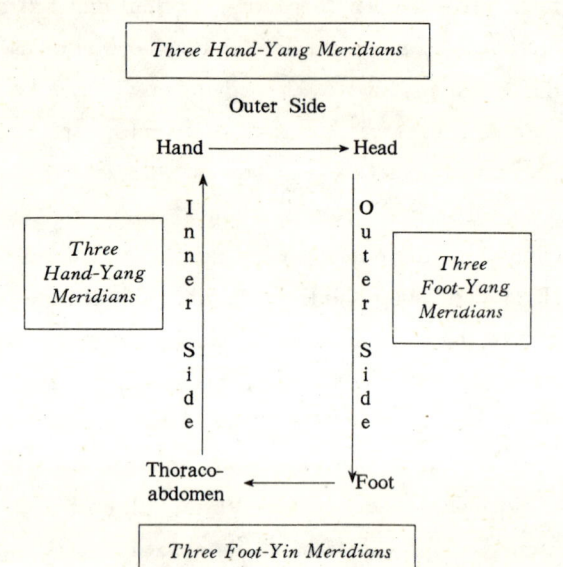

```
           ┌─────────────────────────────┐
           │  Three Hand-Yang Meridians  │
           └─────────────────────────────┘
                      Outer Side
           Hand ──────────────→ Head
                  ↑              │
                  I              O
   ┌──────────┐   n              u   ┌──────────┐
   │  Three   │   n              t   │  Three   │
   │Hand-Yang │   e              e   │Foot-Yang │
   │Meridians │   r              r   │Meridians │
   └──────────┘   S              S   └──────────┘
                  i              i
                  d              d
                  e              e
                  │              ↓
           Thoraco- ←────────── Foot
           abdomen
           ┌─────────────────────────────┐
           │  Three Foot-Yin Meridians   │
           └─────────────────────────────┘
```

Most acupoints are located on the meridians, so they are called "meridian points". Some acupoints are not located on the meridians, but they also have therapeutic effects on certain diseases. Such acupoints are called "extraordinary acupoints", for example, the acupoint Taiyang (Extra). Some locations may show tenderness when there is a disease or are sensitive and effective in a treatment. They are called "Ashi points" or "Tianying points".

Acupoints with beautifying effects are many.

Massaging these acupoints may produce good efficacy on disorders affecting beauty, such as baldness, facial paralysis, acne, dermatitis, poor complexion and obesity.

There are three methods of point selection. One is bonelength measurement, a method to locate acupoints by virtue of the length of equally divided portions of a particular long bone. For example, the distance from the front hairline to the back hairline in the head is 12 *cun*. The length of one cun for any person, either male or female, tall or short, fat or thin, is the same. The second method is identical-unit measurement: the thumb and middle-finger tips are connected to form a ring, and the length of the outer side of the middle section of the middle finger between the transverse creases of the two ends is defined as one cun called "identical cun". The third method is to take the various anatomic indexes on the surface of the human body as the bases for selecting acupoints, for example, the middle point on the vertex where the imaginary lines ascending from the tips of both ears meet is the acupoint Baihui (GV 20). See Figures 2-1, 2-2, 2-3 and 2-4.

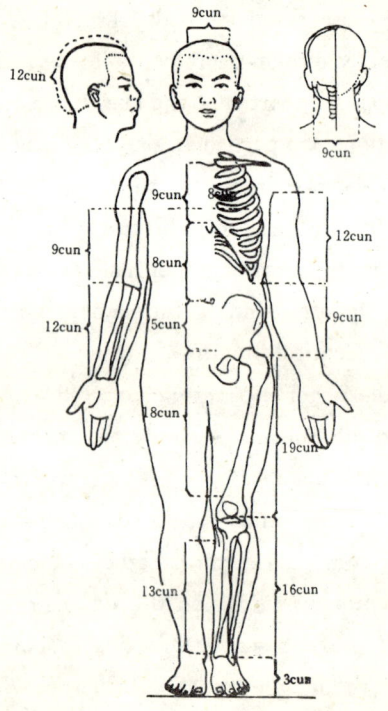

Fig. 2-1 Diagram of common bone-length measurement

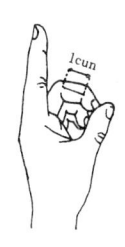

Fig. 2-2
Identical-unit measurement of the middle finger

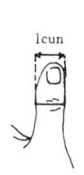

Fig. 2-3
Identical-unit measurement of the thumb

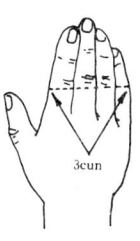

Fig. 2-4
Identical-unit measurement of the horizontal width of the fingers

Table 2-1 Table of the bone-length measurement of the human body

Locations	Starting and ending points	Length
Head	Middle of the front hairline to the middle of the back hairline; Yingtang (Extra) to Naohu (GV 17);	12 cun
	Yintang between the eyebrows to the middle of the front hairline	3 cun
	Spinous process of the 7th cervical vertebra namely Dazhui (GV 14) to the middle of the back hairline	3 cun
	Between the two Wangu (G 12) behind the ears	9 cun

Thoraco-ab-domen	Between the nipples	8 cun
	Lateral thorax, from the transverse crease of the axillary fossa to the 11th costal margin	12 cun
	Upper abdomen, from the inferior margin of the sternum to the umbilical center	8 cun
	Lower abdomen, from the umbilical center to the superior margin of the pubis	5 cun
Back-waist	Hands holding the elbows, from the midline of the spine to the interior margin of the scapula	3 cun
	From Dazhui (GV 14) to coccyx and sacrum	30 cun
Upper extremity	From the end of the transverse crease of the axillary fossa to the transverse crease of the elbow	9 cun
	From the transverse crease of the elbow to the transverse crease of the wrist	12 cun
Lower extremity	Inner side of the thigh, from the place level with the superior margin of the pubis to the medial epicondyle of thigh	18 cun
	Outer side of the thigh, from the greater trochanter of femur to the place level with popliteal transverse crease	19 cun
	Inner side of the shank, from inner condyle of tibia to the tip of medial malleolus	13 cun
	Outer side of the shank, from the place level with the popliteal transverse crease to the tip of lateral malleolus	16 cun

The pathways of the fourteen meridians are determined by the *Yin* or *Yang* properties of the interior organs they connect with respectively and by the parts of the body along which they run. The formula is, "The three Hand-*Yin* meridians run from the chest to the hand, the three Hand-*Yang* meridians run from hand back to the head, the three Foot-*Yang* meridians run from the head to the outer side of the foot, the three Foot-*Yin* meridians run along the inner side of the foot, the Conception Vessel governs *Yin* meridians and runs in the front midline, and the Governor Vessel governs *Yang* meridians and runs in the back midline." The meridians are discussed respectively as follows.

The Lung Meridian of Hand-*Taiyin*.

Running from the chest to the hand, along the anterior margin of the palmar side of the upper extremity. It originates in the middle portion of the body cavity above the diaphragm (the stomach), running downward to the large intestine, turning back, it reaches the stomach and enters the thoracic cavity through an orifice in the diaphragm to enter its pertaining organ, the lung. Running along the trachea it reaches the larynx, then it turns downward and laterally exits at the thoracic cavity below the peripheral portion of the clavicle at acupoint Zhongfu (L 1). Descending along the medial surface of the upper arm along the lateral side of the tendon of the biceps brachii muscle it reaches the cubital fossa. From there it runs on the palmar surface of the forearm toward the radial artery passes the thenar group, enters the thumb ending in acupoint Shaoshang (L 11) in the medial side of the fingernail (Fig. 2-5).

At acupoint Lieque (L 7) a small branch splits from the main meridian and runs along the inner side of the index finger to the tip of the index finger, where it connects with the Large Intestine Meridian of Hand-*Yangming*.

The Large Intestine Meridian of Hand-*Yangming*

Running from the hand to the head, along the anterior margin of the dorsal side of the upper extremity and over the front part of the face. It starts from acupoint Shangyang (LI 1) on the tip of the radial side of the index finger, running upward along the radial side of the index finger, then along the second metacarpal bone, into the depression between tendons of the extensor pollicis longus and brevis muscles, along the anterio-lateral side of the forearm to the lateral side of the elbow. From

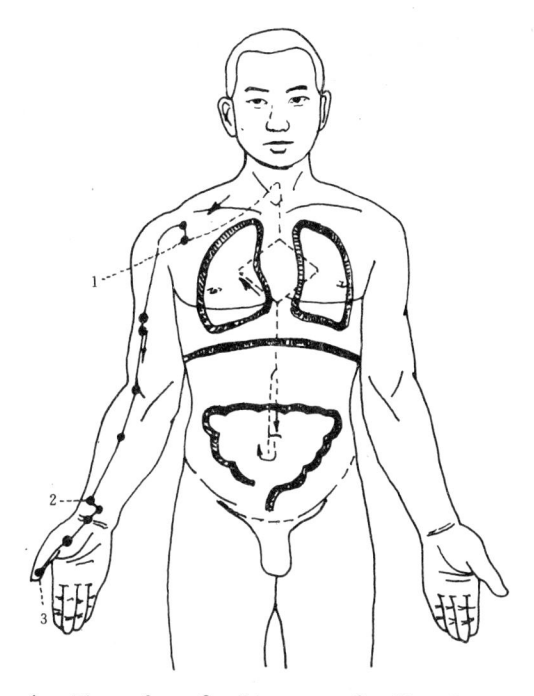

1. *Zhongfu*   2. *Lieque*   3. *Shaoshang*

Fig. 2-5   The Lung Meridian of Hand-*Taiyin*

there it runs along the lateral surface of the arm upward to the shoulder, meets with acupoint Bingfeng (SI 12) of the Small Intestine Meridian, and turns toward the cervical vertebra to acupoint Dazhui (GV 14). It then turns to the supraclavicular fossa, runs downward into the lung, crosses the diaphragm and connects with its pertaining organ, the large intestine (Fig. 2-6). Its branch runs upward from the supraclavicular fossa toward the neck, reaches the cheek, enters the lower gum, turns out and curves around the lips, passes acupoint Renzhong (GV 26), and ends in acupoint Yingxiang (LI 20), where it connects with the Stomach Meridian of Foot-*Yangming*.

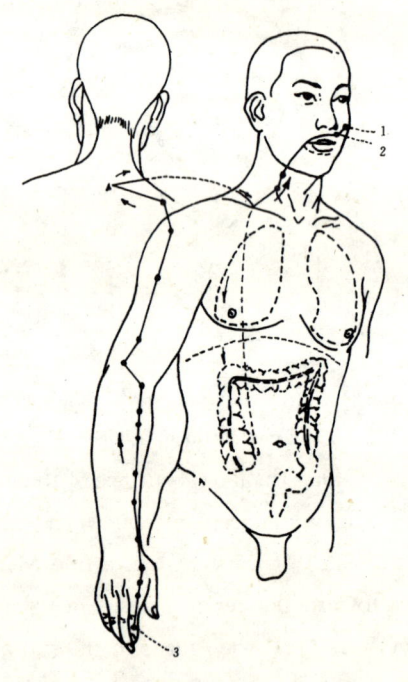

1. *Yingxiang*   2. *Heliao*   3. *Shangyang*
Fig. 2-6   The Large Intestine Meridian of Hand-*Yangming*

The Stomach Meridian of Foot-*Yangming*.

Running from the head to the foot, over the face, along the front of the thoracoabdomen and the anterior margin of the outer side of the lower extremity. This meridian is divided into 6 routes, namely: 1) Meridian from beside the nose to the forehead. This starts from the point between the naso-labial groove and midpoint of nasalala, ascends to base of nose, descending to acupoint Chengqi (ST 1), which is slightly above the inferior border of the eye socket and further down to upper gum. Curving around the lips it joins acupoint Chengjiang (CV 24) under the lower lip, runs along the mandible posteriorly to acupoint Jiache (ST 6), turns upward, past acupoint Shangguan (G 3), along the hairline to the middle of forehead. 2) Branch from the mandible to the abdomen. This descends from acupoint Daying (ST 5) to acupoint Renying (ST 9), runs along the throat to the supraclavicular fossa, enters the thorax cavity and penetrates the diaphragm, runs to the stomach and connects with the spleen. 3) Straight meridian from the supraclavicular fossa to the thoraco-abdomen. This starts from the supraclavicular fossa, passes the nipple, descends to the inguinal canal and joins acupoint Qijie (ST 30).

4) Branch from the stomach to the second toe. From the stomach it descends along the anterior wall of the abdomen to acupoint Qijie (ST 30), runs downward through acupoints Piguan and Futu (ST 32) to the whirbone at the knee. Then it runs along the anteriolateral surface of the cruris to the dorsum of the foot, into the medial side of the middle toe, and ends in acupoint Lidui (ST 45) on the tip of the second toe. 5) Branch from the shank to the middle toe. This splits from the place 3 cun under the knee and descends to the lateral side of the middle toe. 6) Branch from the back of foot to the big toe. This splits from the dorsum of the foot and terminates on the medial side of the big toe, where it connects with the Spleen Meridian of Foot-*Taiyin* (Fig. 2-7).

The Spleen Meridian of Foot-*Taiyin*.

Running from the foot to the thoraco-abdomen, along the anterior margin of the medial side of the lower extremity to the anterior wall of the thoracoabdomen. It starts from acupoint Yinbai (Sp 1) on the medial side of the big toe, runs along the medial side of the big toe, turns upward just before the medial malleolus, then it turns towards the back edge of tibia and meets in front of the Liver Meridian of Foot-*Jueyin* at the location 8

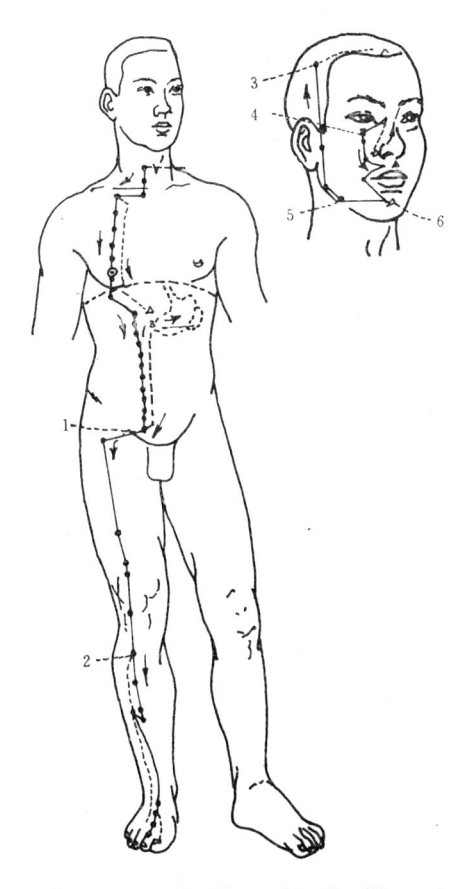

1. *Qichong*   2. *Zusanli*   3. *Touwei*
4. *Chengqi*   5. *Renying*   6. *Chengjiang*

Fig. 2-7 The Stomach Meridian of Foot-*Taiyang*

cun above the medial malleolus. It then passes through the anterior medial aspect of the knee and thigh and traveling further upward across the abdomen enters the abdominal cavity, the spleen, its pertaining organ and the stomach. It then transverses the diaphragm traveling along the esophagus to the base of the tongue and branches out under the tongue (Fig. 2-8). Its branch deviates from the stomach and runs upward, transverses the diaphragm and enters the heart, where it connects with the Heart Meridian of Hand-*Shaoyin*.

The Heart Meridian of Hand-*Shaoyin*.

Running from the chest to the hand, along the posterior border of the palmar side of the upper extremity. It ascends from the heart, passes the lung to the inferior aspect of the axillary fossa, runs along the posterior border of the medial surface of upper extremity to the posterior aspect of the Lung Meridian of Hand-*Taiyin* and the Pericardium Meridian of Hand-*Jueyin*, descends to the medial side of the cubital fossa, runs along the posterior border of the medial side of the forearm into the posterior border of the medial side of the palm, and ends at acupoint Shaochong (H 9) at the tip of the little finger, where it connects with the Small Intestine Meridian of Hand-*Taiyang* (Fig. 2-9). It has two branches: 1) Starts from

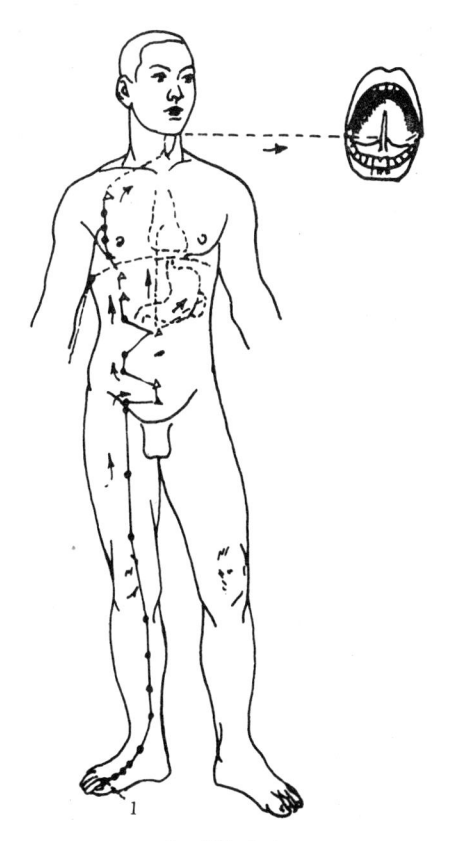

1. *Yinbai*

Fig. 2-8 The Spleen Meridian of Foot-*Taiyin*

the heart, runs downward, crosses the diaphragm and enters the small intestine. 2) Starts from the heart, runs upward along the esophagus, pharynx and joins the meridians in back of the eyeball.

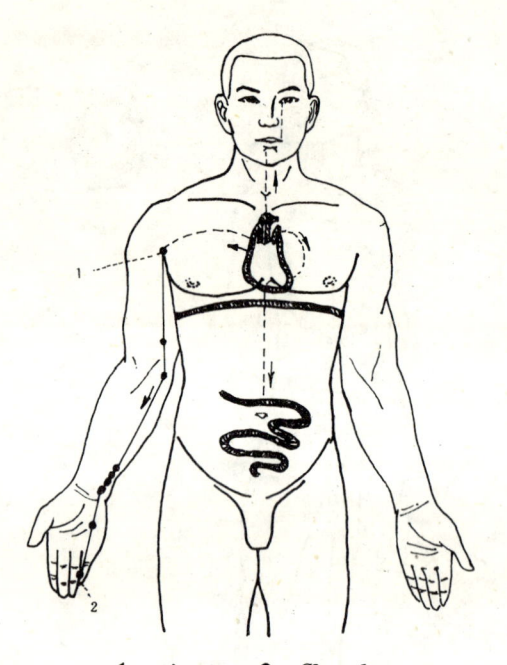

1. *Jiquan*　2. *Shaochong*

Fig. 2-9　The Heart Meridian of Hand-*Shaoyin*

The small Intestine Meridian of Hand-*Taiyang*.

This runs from the hand to the head, along the posterior border of the dorsal side of upper extremity, over the cheek to the anteriority of the ear. It starts from acupoint Shaoze (SI 1) on the ulnar side of the tip of the little finger, ascends along the lateral side of the hand to the wrist, passes the styloid process of the ulna, runs upward along the posterior border of the dorsal side of the forearm, passes through between the ulnar olecranoid process of elbow joint and medial epicondyle of the humerus, then runs upward along the posterior border of the lateral side of the arm to the shoulder joint, from whence it transverses the scapula, goes over the shoulder, turns downward into the supraclavicular fossa; descending into the heart, it runs along the esophagus, crosses the diaphragm, enters the stomach and runs down to connect with the small intestine (Fig. 2-10). It has two branches: 1) Ascending from the supraclavicular fossa, it runs along the neck to the cheek, reaches the external canthus, turns back to the ear and ends at acupoint Tinggong (SI 19). 2) Splitting from the cheek, it ascends to under the orbit, runs along the nose to the inner canthus and connects with the Bladder Meridian of Foot-*Taiyang*.

The Bladder Meridian of Foot-*Taiyang*.

This runs from the head to the foot, along the vertex, the nape of the neck, the back and the midline of the posterior side of the lower extremity. This meridian is divided into 5 routes, namely: 1) Starting from acupoint Jingming (B 1) near the inner corner of the eye, it runs upward, passes the forehead and ascends to the vertex. 2)

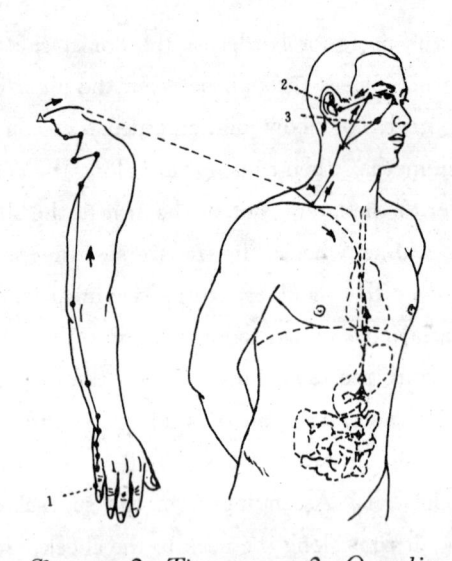

1. *Shaoze* 2. *Tinggong* 3. *Quanliao*

Fig. 2-10   The Small Intestine Meridian of Hand-
Taiyang

Starting from the vertex and running horizontally to above the auricular process. 3) Starting from the vertex, it enters the brain, curves out to the top, runs along the medial side of the shoulder and arm, where it bifurcates, one trunk running 1.5 cun from the vertebral column, the other 3 cun from the same line. It runs downward to the waist, enters the kidney, runs forward and connects with the urinary bladder. 4) Starting from the waist, runs downward parallel to the vertebral column, it passes the buttock and enters the popliteal fossa. 5) On the medial side of the shoulder and arm, 3 cun from the vertebral column, it passes the interior border of the scapula, runs downward parallel to the vertebral column, passes the greater trochanter, descends along the postero-lateral side of the thigh to the popliteal fossa, where it joins the previous route. It then continues to descend, runs down the posterior side of shank, turns out to the posterior border of the external malleolus, passes the acupoint Jinggu (B 64), and runs along the external side of the foot and ends at acupoint Zhiyin (B 67) on the external side of the little toe, where it connects with the Kidney Meridian of Foot-*Shaoyin* (Fig. 2-11).

The Kidney Meridian of Foot-*Shaoyin*.

This runs from the foot to the thoraco-abdomen, along the posterior border of the internal side of lower extremity to the anterior side of the thoraco-abdomen. It starts from under the little toes, runs obliquely to the center of the sole, passes acupoint Rangu (K 2), turns toward the tuberosity of the navicular bone running behind it to the medial malleolus, enters the heel and runs upward to connects with the Spleen Meridian of Foot-*Taiyin* at acupoint Sanyinjiao (Sp 6); it then ascends along the medial side of the popliteal

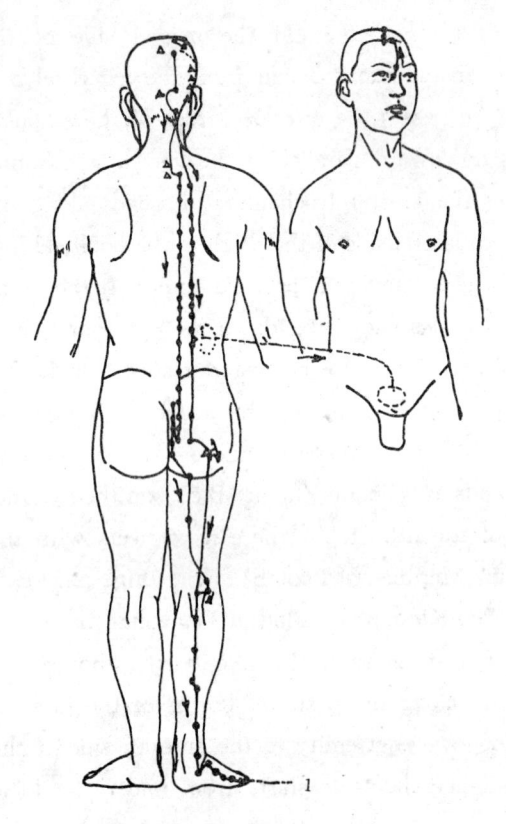

1. *Zhiyin*

Fig. 2-11 The Bladder Meridian of Foot-*Taiyang*

fossa to the posterior aspect of the medial side of the thigh and joins the Governor Vessel at acupoint Changqiang (GV 1). Next it runs along the spinal column to the kidney and enters the urinary bladder, where it connects with the Governor Vessel at acupoints Guanyuan (CV 4) and Zhongji (CV 3) (Fig. 2-12). It has two branches: 1) Ascending from the kidney, it passes the liver and diaphragm and enters the lung and trachea, then ends at the base of the tongue. 2) Branching from the lung, it enters the pericardium, and spreads throughout the chest.

The Pericardium Meridian of Hand-*Jueyin*.

Running from the chest to the hand, along the midline of the palmar side of upper extremity. It commences in the chest where it connects with its pertaining organ the pericardium. It then descends through the diaphragm into the abdomen, linking with the Triple Energizer Meridian. Its branch runs from the chest to the intercostal space, emerges in acupoint Tianchi (P 1) located inferiorly and laterally from the the nipple and reaches the axillary fossa. The branch then runs along the medial surface of the upper arm between the Lung meridian of Hand-*Taiyin* and the Heart Meridian of Hand-*Shaoyin*, passes the elbow joint and descends in between the tendons of palmaris longus and flexor carpi radialis muscles to the palm and reaches acupoint Zhongchong (P 9) at the tip of the middle finger (Fig. 2-13). Its branch divides off in the palm and runs to the tip of the ring fin-

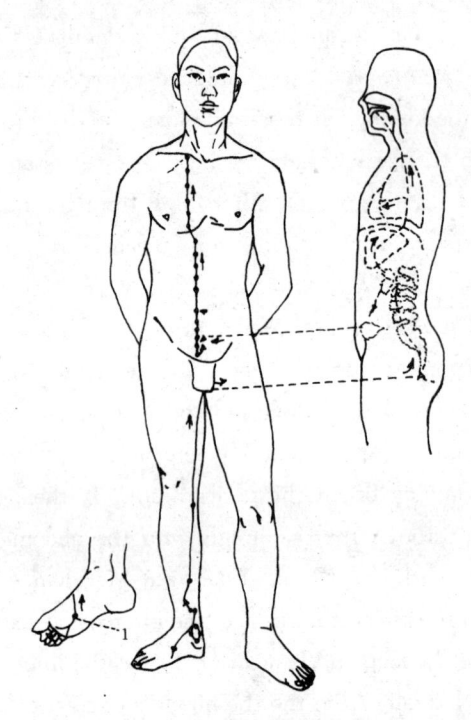

1. *Yongquan*

Fig. 2-12　The Kidney Meridian of Foot-*Shaoyin*

ger, where it connects with the Triple Energizer Meridian of Hand-*Shaoyang*.

The Triple Energizer Meridian of Hand-*Shaoyang*.

This runs from the hand to the head, along the midline of the dorsal side of upper extremity to exterior border of the ear. It originates from the

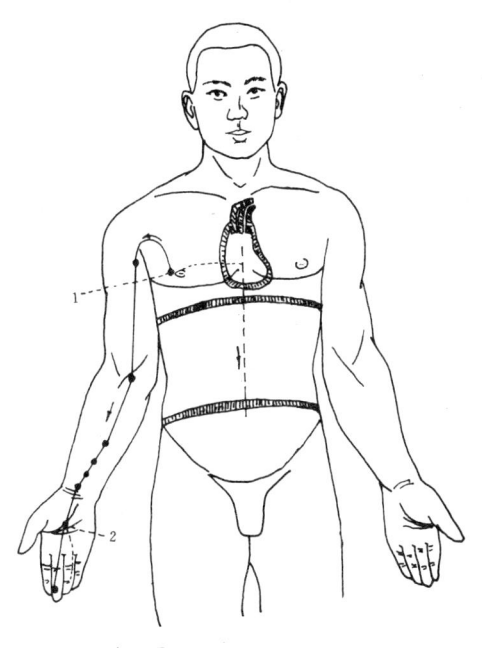

1. *Tianchi*   2. *Laogong*

Fig. 2-13   The Pericardium Meridian of Hand-*Jueyin*

ulnar side of the tip of the ring finger, runs between the 4th and 5th metacarpal bones up the dorsal side of the wrist, then along the dorsal side of the forearm between the radius and ulna to the olecranon, passing it laterally; reaching the shoulder region, it connects with the Small Intestine Meridian of Hand-*Taiyang* at acupoint Bingfeng (SI 12), connects with the Governor Vessel at acupoint Dazhui (GV 14), connects with the Gallbladder Meridian of Foot-*Shaoyang* at acupoint Jianjing (G 21), and reaches the supraclavicular fossa. It then passes acupoint Shanzhong (CV 17), transverses the diaphragm and enters the abdomenal cavity, connecting the upper, middle and lower warmers (Fig. 2-14).

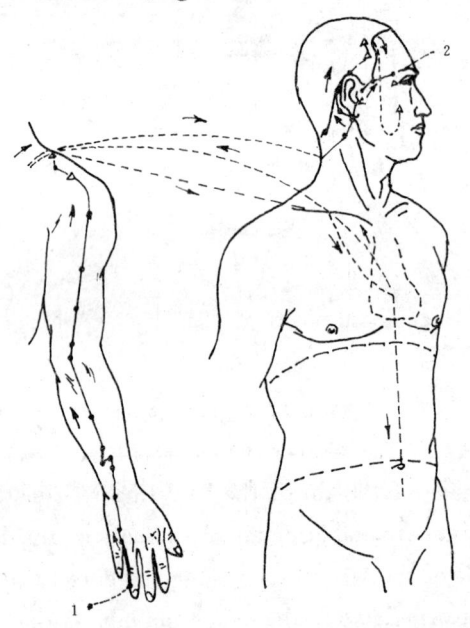

1. *Guanchong* 2. *Sizhukong*

Fig. 2-14 The Triple Energizer Meridian of Hand-*Shaoyang*

Branches: 1) Ascending from acupoint Shanzhong (CV 17), it passes the supraclavicular fossa, runs along the lateral surface of the neck, along the posterior part of the ear, connects with the Gallbladder Meridian of Foot-*Shaoyang* at acupoints Xuanli (G 6) and Hanyan (G 4), then descends to the cheek, and terminates in the infraorbital region, where it connects with the Small Intestine Meridian of Hand-*Taiyang* at acupoint Quanliao (SI 18). 2) Originating from behind the ear, it enters the ear, emerges in front of it, connects with the Small Intestine Meridian of Hand-*Taiyang* at acupoint Tinggong (SI 19), passes in front of acupoint Shangguan (G 3), runs to the cheek, reaches the extra-ocular region and terminates at acupoint Sizhukong (TE 23), where it connects with the Gallbladder Meridian of Foot-*Shaoyang*.

The Gallbladder Meridian of Foot-*Shaoyang*.

This runs from the head to the foot, along the lateral side of the head and the midline of the external side of lower extremity (Fig. 2-15).

This meridian is divided into 5 routes: 1) Emerging from acupoint Tongziliao (G 1), which is near the external corner of the eye, it ascends to the forehead angle, curves around the lateral side of the head, turns behind and below to circle the auricula, runs along the nape of the neck and in front

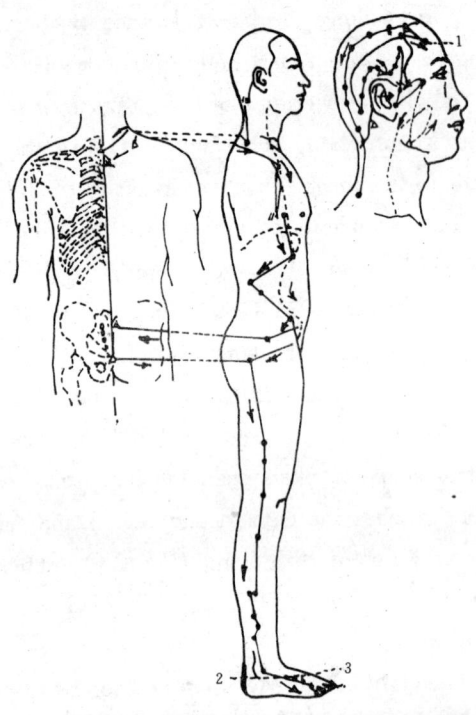

1. *Yangbai* 2. *Zulingi* 3. *Zuqiaoyin*
Fig. 2-15 The Gallbladder Meridian of Foot-*Shaoyang*

of the Triple Energizer Meridian of Hand-*Shaoyang* to the shoulder, then runs to the back of the Triple Energizer Meridian and enters acupoint Quepen (S 12). 2) Starting from the back of the ear, it enters the ear, re-emerges from the ear and reaches the location outside the outer canthus. 3) Branching from the corner of the outer

96

canthus, it descends to acupoint Daying (S 5) of the Stomach Meridian of Foot-*Yangming* and connects with the Triple Energizer Meridian of Hand-*Shaoyang*. From here it reaches the inferior border of the orbit, passes the mandible and descends to acupoint Quepen (S 12); running further down, it enters the thoracic cavity, crosses the diaphragm, and enters the liver and its pertaining organ the gallbladder. From there it descends along the costa to acupoint Qichong (S 30). After curving around the pudendum, it emerges and joins acupoint Huantiao (G 30). 4) Emerging from acupoint Quepen (S 12), it runs down to the axillary fossa, passes the chest and enters acupoint Huantiao (G 30). It then runs further down along the lateral side of the knee and the anterior border of the fibula to the lower end of os fibula 3 cun above the lateral malleolus, runs in front of the lateral malleolus to the dorsum of the foot and ends at acupoint Qiaoyin (G 44) at the external tip of the 4th toe. 5) Deviating from the dorsum of the foot, it runs along the crevice between the metatarsal bones of the big and second toes to the tip of the big toe, where it connects with the Liver Meridian of Foot-*Jueyin*.

The Liver Meridian of Foot-*Jueyin*.

This runs from the foot to the thoraco-abdomen, along the midline of the the internal side of lower extremity and the lateral side of the thoraco-abdomen. It emerges from acupoint Dadun (Liv 1), which is located on the dorsum of the toe, runs upward along the dorsum of the foot and reaches a point 1 cun in front of the medial malleolus, ascends to a point 8 cun above the medial malleolus, crosses the Spleen Meridian of Foot-*Taiyin*, ascends along the medial side of the knee and thigh to the pubic region where it curves around the external genitalia to the lower abdomen, runs around the stomach and enters the liver and gall bladder. Further on it crosses the diaphragm, passes the hypochondrium, ascends along the posterior aspect of the throat, through the plate , and connects with the meridians in back of the eyeball. It then runs further upward to the forehead and meets on the vertex with the Governor Vessel (Fig. 2-16). It has two branches: 1) Originating from the meridians in back of the eyeball, it runs downwards to the cheek and curves around the inner surface of the lips. 2) Emerging from the liver, it transverses the diaphragm, ascends into the lung and connects with the Lung Meridian of Hand-*Taiyin*.

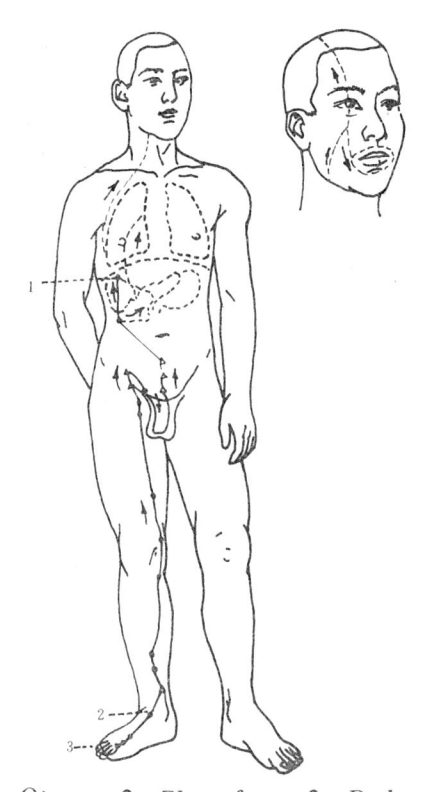

1. *Qimen* 2. *Zhongfeng* 3. *Dadun*

Fig. 2-16 The Liver Meridian of Foot-*Jueyin*

The Governor Vessel.

This begins in the belly and descends to the perineum; ascending from acupoint Changqiang (GV 1) along the middle of the spinal column, it passes acupoint Fengfu (GV 16), enters the brain and ascends to the vertex of the head, after which it descends to the forehead along the middle of which it runs to the tip of the nose, then ends at acupoint Yinjiao (GV 28) in the upper lip (Fig. 2-17). The Governor Vessel governs the *Yang* meridians of the entire body, so it is referred to as the "sea of *yang* meridians".

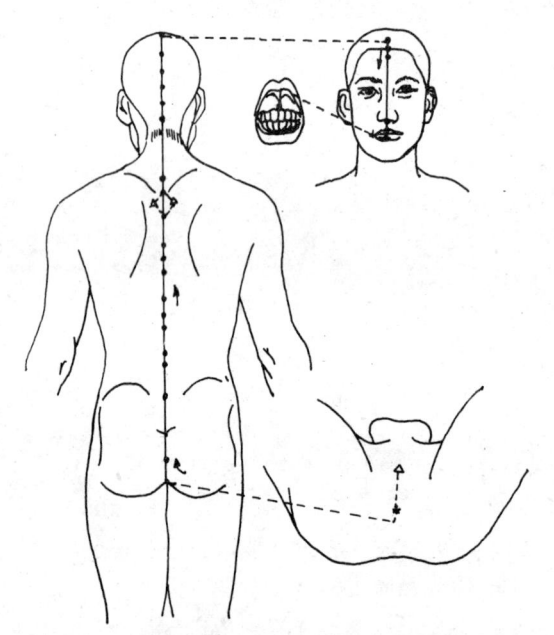

Fig. 2-17 The Governor Vessel

The Conception Vessel.

This starts from the pelvic cavity and emerges at the perineum, then runs anteriorly across the pubic region and ascends along the midline of the abdomen through acupoint Guanyuan (CV 4) up to the throat and lower cheek, curving around the lips and ending at the inferior border of the orbit (Fig. 2-18). Running along the abdomen and connecting with all the *Yin* meridians, the Conception Vessel is the key link of *yin* meridians, so it is referred to as the "sea of *yin* meridians".

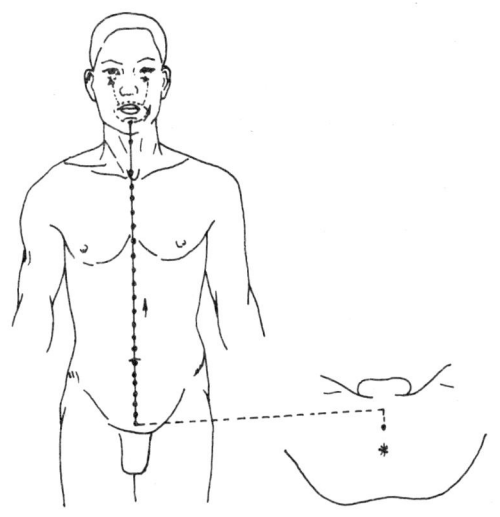

Fig. 2-18 The Conception Vessel

Among the fourteen meridians, the running laws of the Twelve Meridians are: The three hand-*yin* meridians run from the chest to the hand; the three hand-*yang* meridians run from the hand to the head; the three foot-*yang* meridians run from the foot to the head; and the three foot-*yin* meridians run from the foot to the chest (abdomen).

The selection of acupoints and selection of supporting acupoints may abide by the principles of proximity, extremity, anteriority and posteriority according to their indications and pertaining meridians.

For common acupoints, see the following table:

Table 2-2 Common Acupoints and Their Indications and Beautifying Effects

I. The Lung Meridian of the Hand-*Taiyin*
ACUPOINTS, LOCATIONS AND INDICATIONS:
1. Zhoungfu (L 1): located 6 cun laterally to the front midline, parallel with the 1st intercostal space.

Indications: cought, asthma, back or shoulder pain.

2. Chize (L 5): located in the cubital crease on the radial side of the tendon of biceps brachii muscle.

Indications: spasmodic pain of elbow and arm, cough, asthma, fullness in the chest and hypochondrium, infantile convulsion.

3. Kongzui (L 6): located on the radial side of the forearm on the line connecting Chize (L 5) and Taiyuan (L 9), 7

cun above the transverse crease of the wrist.

Indications: cought, hemoptysis, hoarseness, sore-throat, elbowpain.

4. Lieque (L 7): located above the the styloid process of the radius, 1.5 cun above the transverse crease of the wrist.

Indications: cought, short breath, rigidity of nape with headache, toothache.

5. Taiyuan (L 9): located on the palmar surface at the tip of the transverse crease of the wrist, in the depression on the radial side of the radial artery.

Indications: Cough, asthma, mammary swelling, sore throat, wrist pain.

6. Yuji (L 10): located in the middle of the 1st metacarpal bone, on the dorso-ventral boundary of the hand.

Indications: chest and back pain, headache, dizziness, laryngalgia, fever with chills.

7. Shaoshang (L 11): located on the radial side of the thumb, approximately 0.1 cun from the corner of the nail.

Indications: apoplectic coma, spasm of fingers, infantile convulsion.

BEAUTIFYING EFFECTS:

Helping prevent and treat exopathic diseases, supplementing lung qi, and treating roughness of complexion, brandy nose, edema and other dermatoses.

Ⅱ. The Large Intestine Meridian of Hand-*Yangming*
ACUPOINTS, LOCATIONS AND INDICATIONS:

1. Hegu (LI 4): located between the 1st and 2nd metacarpal bones on the dorsum, roughly parallel with the middle of the 2nd metacarpal bone.

Indications: headache, toothache, fever, laryngalgia, spasm of finger, arm pain, facial paralysis.

2. Yangxi (LI 5): located on the radial side of the dorsal transverse crease of the wrist, between the two tendons.

Indications: headache, tinnitus, toothache, swelling and sore throat, conjunctival congestion, wrist pain.

3. Pianli (LI 6): located on the line connecting Yangxi (LI 5) and Quchi (LI 11), 3 cun above Yangxi (LI 5).

Indications: epistaxis, conjunctival congestion, tinnitus, soreness and pain of hand and arm, laryngalgia, edema.

4. Wenliu (LI 7): located on the line connecting Yangxi (LI 5) and Quchi (LI 11), 5 cun above Yangxi (LI 5).

Indications: Abdominal pain, hiccup, throat and tongue pain, headache.

5. Shousanli (LI 10): located 2 cun under Quchi (LI 11).

Indications: elbow spasm, difficulty in bending and extending, numbness, soreness and pain of arm.

6. Quchi (LI 11): located in the depression on the frontolateral side of the transverse crease of the elbow when the elbow is bent.

Indications: fever, hypertension, swelling and pain of arm, elbow pain, upper extremity paralysis.

7. Jianyu (LI 15): located on lateral surface of arm, inferiorly and posteriorly from acromion. Best seen when arm

is raised, in a depression on the anterior skin crest.

Indications: shoulder pain, disturbances in the movement of shoulder joints, paralysis.

8. Yingxiang (LI 20): located 0.5 cun laterally to the wing of nost, in the naso-labial groove.

Indications: rhinitis, nasal obstruction, facial paralysis

BEAUTIFYING EFFECTS:

Treating constipation and skin rash, preventing and treating diarrhea, and also effective on leptochroa, deafness and blurring of vision, cheek edema, conjunctival congestion, ophthalmalgia and toothache; improving dim complexion.

III. The Stomach Meridian of Foot-*Yangming*

ACUPOINTS, LOCATIONS AND INDICATIONS:

1. Sibai (S 2): located directly under the pupil when one looks straight ahead, below inferior edge of eyesocket, in the depression of the infraorbital foramen.

Indications: facial paralysis, conjunctival congestion, eye pain and itching.

2. Dicang (S 4): located 0.4 cun laterally from corner of mouth.

Indications: salivation, facial paralysis.

3. Daying (S 5): located in the bone lacuna 1.3 cun in front of the angle of mandible.

Indications: lockjaw, toothache.

4. Jiache (S 6): located in the depression a finger-diameter's width above and anterior to jaw angle at the prominence of masseter muscle.

Indications: facial paralysis, toothache, cheek edema.
5. Xiaguan (S 7): located in the depression below zygomatic arch, anteriorly to condyloid process of mandible.

Indications: facial paralysis, toothache.
6. Touwei (S 8): located 0.5 cun directly above the hairline of forehead angle.

Indications: headache.
7. Renying (S 9): located 1.5 cun laterally to the laryngeal protuberance.

Indications: swelling and soreness of throat, asthma, scrofula, nape edema, dyspnea.
8. Shuitu (S 10): located 1 cun below Renying (S 9), on the anterior border of sternocleidomastoid muscle.

Indications: fullness sensation in chest, cough, stiffness of nape.
9. Quepen (S 12): located in the center of the supraclavicular fossa, 4 cun laterally to the front midline.

Indications: fullness sensation in chest, cough, stiffness of nape.
10. Tianshu (S 25): located 2 cun laterally to umbilicus.

Indications: diarrhea, constipation, abdominal pain, irregular menstruation.
11. Biguan (S 31): located on the line connecting the anterior superior iliac crest and the exterior border of the patella, parallel with the gluteal groove.

Indications: pain in waist and lower extremities, lower extremity numbness, flaccidity and lassitude, muscular spasm and contracture, difficulty in bending and extending.

12. Futu (ST 32): located 6 cun above the exterior and superior border of the patella.

Indications: pain, coldness and numbness of the knee, paralysis of lower extremities.

13. Liangqiu (S 34): located 2 cun above the exterior and superior border of the patella.

Indications: knee pain, coldness and numbness.

14. Dubi (S 35): located in the depression on the inferior border of the patella, lateral to patellar ligament.

Indications: soreness, pain and difficult activity of knee joint.

15. Zusanli (S 36): located 3 cun below Dubi (S 35), a fingerdiameter's width laterally to anterior tibial crest.

Indications: abdominal pain, diarrhea, constipation, coldness and numbness of lower extremities, hypertension.

16. Shangjuxu (S 37): located 3 cun below Zusanli (S 36).

Indications: abdominal pain, diarrhea, paralysis of lower extremities.

17. Xiajuxu (S 39): located 3 cun below Shangjuxu (S 37).

Indications: belly pain, pain along spinal column, acute mastitis, flaccidity of lower extremities.

18. Fenglong (S 40): located at the midpoint of the line connecting Dubi (S 35) and the tip of lateral malleolus.

Indications: headache, productive cough, edema of extremities, constipation, epilepsy, flaccidity of lower extremities.

19. Jiexi (S 41): located at the midpoint of the transverse crease of the ankle joint on the dorsum of foot, between tendon extensor digitorum longus and hallucis longus muscles.

Indications: sprain of the ankle joint, numbness of foot and toe.

20. Chongyang (S 42): located 1.5 cun below Jiexi (S 41), the highest point of the dorsum of foot, where the artery can be felt.

Indications: facial paralysis, facial edema, pain of upper teeth, stomachache, paralysis of foot muscles, epilepsy.

BEAUTIFYING EFFECTS:

Improving pathologic leanness, promoting the development of mammary glands, treating aphthae, facial paralysis, pathologic leanness, polyorexia, insomnia and dyspepsia; certain therapeutic effects on skin rash and sallow and dim skin.

Ⅳ. The Spleen Meridian of Foot-*Taiyin*

ACUPOINTS, LOCATIONS AND INDICATIONS:

1. Taibai (Sp 3): located at the posterior border of the capitulum of the lst metatarsal bone, on the dorso-ventral boundary of the hand.

Indications: stomachache, abdominal distention, borborygmus, diarrhea, constipation, hemorrhoid complicated by anal fistula.

2. Gongsun (Sp 4): located at the anterior border of the

base of the lst metatarsal bone, on the dorso-ventral boundary of the hand.

Indications: stomachache, vomiting, dyspepsia, abdominal pain, diarrhea, dysentery.

3. Sanyinjiao (Sp 5): located 3 cun above the medial malleolus, in the center of the the medial side of the tibia.

Indications: insomnia, abdominal distention, lack of appetite, enuresis, difficulty in micturition, gynecological disorders.

4. Diji (Sp 8): located 3 cun below Yinlingquan (Sp 9).

Indications: abdominal pain, diarrhea, edema, difficulty in micturition, nocturnal ejaculation.

5. Yinlingquan (Sp 9): located in the depression on the inferior border of the medial condyle of the tibia.

Indications: soreness and pain of knee joint, difficulty in micturition.

6. Xuehai (Sp 10): located 2 cun above the internal angle of the patella.

Indications: irregular menstruation, knee pain.

7. Daheng (Sp 15): located 4 cun laterally to umbilicus.

Indications: diarrhea or dysentery due to cold of insufficiency type, constipation, belly pain.

BEAUTIFYING EFFECTS:

Preventing pathologic leanness, losing weight, eliminating edema, treating epigastraligia, loose stool, dyspepsia, sallow complexion, roughness of skin fatigue, liability to tiredness, and various kinds of bleeding symptoms.

V. The Heart Meridian of Hand-*Shaoyin*

ACUPOINTS, LOCATIONS AND INDICATIONS:

1. Jiquan (H 1): located in the center of the axillary fossa.

Indications: choking sensation in chest, costalgia, coldness and numbness of arm and elbow.

2. Shaohai (H 3): located in the depression at the end of the ulnar side of the transverse crease of elbow when the elbow is bent.

Indications: pain of elbow joint, twitch of hand and spasm of elbow.

3. Tongli (H 5): located 1 cun above Shenmen (H 7).

Indications: heart palpitation, severe palpitation, dizziness, pharyngodynia, sudden loss of voice, stiff tongue and loss of voice, wrist and arm pain.

4. Yinxi (H 6): located 0.5 cun above Shenmen (H 7).

Indications: heart pain, heart palpitation, hectic fever and night sweat, hematemesis, hemoptysis, sudden loss of voice.

5. Shenmen (H 7): located on the ulnar side of the transverse crease of wrist, on the radial side of pasiform bone in the depression of the radial side of the tendon of flexor carpi ulnaris muscle.

Indications: heart palpitation, severe palpitation, insomnia, amnesia.

BEAUTIFYING EFFECTS:

Treating neurosism, heart palpitation, insomnia, restlessness, pale complexion, pale or dark purple nail, and relieving fatigue and emotional excitement.

Ⅵ. The Small Intestine Meridian of Hand-*Taiyang*
ACUPOINTS, LOCATIONS AND INDICATIONS:

1. Shaoze (SI 1): located about 0.1 cun by the corner of nail at ulnar side of small finger.

Indications: fever, apoplectic coma, hypogalactia, throat swelling and pain.

2. Houxi (SI 3): located on posterior ulnar side of the 5th metacarpophalangeal joint, at the head of the transverse crease, on the dorso-ventral boundary of the hand.

Indications: rigidity and pain of the nape of neck, deafness, pharyngodynia, toothache, conjunctivitis, spasm and pain of elbow and arm.

3. Wangu (SI 4): located on the ulnar side of the dorsum of hand, in the depression in front of the pisiform bone.

Indications: headache, spasm and pain of shoulder and arm, wrist pain, finger spasm, jaundice, febrile disease without sweat.

4. Yanglao (SI 6): located in the depression on the radial lateral border of the capitulum of ulna.

Indications: failing eyesinght, pain in shoulder, arm and waist.

5. Zhizheng (SI 7): located 5 cun above the wrist, on the dorsal ulnar side of forearm.

Indications: rigidity of nape of neck, spasm of finger, headache, dizziness.

6. Xiaohai (SI 8): located when the elbow is bent in the depression between the olecranon and tip of medial epi-

condyle of the humerus.

Indications: toothache, neck pain, soreness and pain of upper extremities.

7. Jianzhen (SI 9): 1 cun above posterior axillary fold.

Indications: soreness and pain of shoulder joint, difficult activity of shoulder joint, paralysis of upper extremities.

8. Tianzong (SI 11): located in the center of the infraspinous fossa of scapula.

Indications: soreness and pain of shoulder and back, difficult activity of shoulder joint, neck rigidity.

9. Bingfeng (SI 12): located in the supraspinous fossa of scapula.

Indications: scapula pain, impossibility to raise the arm, soreness and numbness of upper extremities.

10. Jianwaishu (SI 14): 3 cun laterally and below the spinous process of lst thoracic vertebra.

Indications: Soreness and pain in shoulder and back, rigidity and spasm of the neck, cold and pain of upper extremities.

11. Jianzhougshu (SI 15): located 2 cun laterally to Dazhui (GV 14).

Indications: cough, asthma, pain of shoulder and back, blurring of vision.

12. Quanliao (SI 18): located directly below the outer canthus, in the depression at the inferior border of the zygomatoid bone.

Indications: facial paralysis.

BEAUTIFYING EFFECTS:

Similar to those of the Large Intestine Meridian of Hand-*Yangming*.

Ⅷ. The Bladder Meridian of Foot-*Taiyang*
ACUPOINTS, LOCATIONS AND INDICATIONS:
1. Jingming (B 1): located 0.1 cun laterally to the inner canthus.

Indications: eye disorders.

2. Zanzhu (B 2): located in the depression at the end of eyebrow.

Indications: headache, insomnia, pain in the supra-orbital bone.

3. Tianzhu (B 10): located 1.3 cun laterally to Yamen (GV 15), in the depression at the exterior border or the trapezius muscle.

Indications: headache, nape rigidity, nasal obstruction, pain of shoulder and back.

4. Dashu (B 11): located 1.5 cun laterally and below the spinous process of the lst thoracic vertebra.

Indications: fever, cough, nape rigidity, soreness and pain of scapula.

5. Fengmen (B 12): located 1.5 cun laterally and inferiorly to the spinous process of the 2nd thoracic vertebra.

Indications: common cold, cough, nape rigidity, pain of waist and back.

6. Feishu (B 13): located 1.5 cun laterally and inferiorly to the spinous process of the 3rd thoracic vertebra.

Indications: cough, asthma, choking sensation in chest,

strain of the muscles of back.

7. Xinshu (B 15): located 1.5 cun laterally and inferiorly to the spinous process of the 5th thoracic vertebra.

Indications: insomnia, heart palpitation.

8. Geshu (B 17): located 1.5 cun laterally and inferiorly to the spinous process of the 7th thoracic vertebra.

Indications: vomition, dysphagia, asthma, cough, night sweats.

9. Ganshu (B 18): located 1.5 cun laterally and inferiorly to the spinous process of the 9th thoracic vertebra.

Indications: pain in hypochondrium, hepatitis, blurring of vision.

10. Danshu (B 19): located 1.5 cun laterally and inferiorly to the spinous process of the 10th thoracic vertebra.

Indications: pain in hypochondrium, bitter taste in the mouth, jaundice.

11. Pishu (B 20): located 1.5 cun laterally and inferiorly to the spinous process of the 11th thoracic vertebra.

Indications: gastric distention and pain, dyspepsia, chronic infantile convulsion.

12. Weishu (B 21): located 1.5 cun laterally and below the spinous process of the 12th thoracic vertebra.

Indications: gastric disorders, infantile vomiting of milk, dyspepsia.

13. Sanjiaoshu (B 22): located 1.5 cun laterally and below the spinous process of the 1st lumbar vertebra.

Indications: borborymus, abdominal distention, vomiting, rigidity and pain of waist and back.

14. Shenshu (B 23): located 1.5 cun laterally and inferiorly to the spinous process of the 2nd lumbar vertebra.

Indications: deficiency of the kidney, lumbago, nocturnal ejaculation, irregular menstruation.

15. Qihaishu (B 24): located 1.5 cun laterally and inferiorly to the spinous process of the 3rd lumbar vertebra.

Indications: lumbago.

16. Dachangshu (B 25): located 1.5 cun laterally and inferiorly to the spinous process of the 4th lumbar vertebra.

Indications: pain in waist and lower extremities, lumbar muscle strain, enteritis.

17. Guanyuanshu (B 26): located 1.5 cun laterally and inferiorly to the spinous process of the 5th lumbar vertebra.

Indications: lumbago, diarrhea.

18. Baliao (B 34): located in the 1st, 2nd, 3rd and 4th posterior sacral foramen (called upper-liao, second-liao, middle-liao and lower-liao respectively).

Indications: pain in waist and lower extremities, disorders in the urinary system.

19. Zhibian (B 54): located 3 cun laterally and inferiorly to the spinous process of the 4th sacral vertebra.

Indications: pain in waist and buttock, flaccidity of lower extremities, urinary incontinence, constipation.

20. Yinmen (B 37): 6 cun below the center of the gluteal groove.

Indications: sciatica, paralysis of lower extremities, pain in waist and back.

21. Weiyang (B 39): located at the external end of the popliteal transverse crease, at the medial border of tendon biceps femoris.

Indications: rigidity and pain of waist and spine, distention in belly, urinary incontinence, spasm and pain of leg and foot.

22. Weizhong (B 40): in the center of the transverse crease of popliteal fossa.

Indications: lumbago, difficult activity of knee joint, hemiparalysis.

23. Chengshan (B 57): located on the top of the depression between the two bellies of gastrocnemius muscle.

Indications: pain in waist an lower extremities, spasm of gastrocnemius muscle.

24. Feiyang (B 58): located 7 cun directly above Kunlun (B 60).

Indications: headache, pain in waist and back, weakness of leg.

25. Fuyang (B 59): located 3 cun directly above Kunlun (B 60).

Indications: headache, lumbar and sacral pain, swelling and pain of lateral malleolus, paralysis of lower extremities.

26. Kunlun (B 60): located in the depression between lateral malleolus and Achilles tendon.

Indications: headache, nape rigidity, lumbago, sprain of ankle joint.

27. Shenmai (B 62): located in the depression at the inferior border of the lateral malleolus.

Indications: epilepsy, pain in waist and lower extremities.
28. Jinmen (B 63): located anteriorly and inferiorly to Shenmen (B 62), in the depression on the lateral side of cuboid bone.

Indications: epilepsy, lumbago, pain of lateral malleolus, pain of lower extremities.
29. Jinggu (B 64): located below tuberosity of the 5th metatarsal bone on the lateral edge of the foot.

Indications: epilepsy, headache, nape rigidity, pain in waist and lower extremities, knee pain, foot spasm.

BEAUTIFYING EFFECTS:

Improving obesity, leptochroa, irregular menstruation, menstrual irritability, endocrine dysfunction, freckles resulting from hypoplasia of uterus, butterfly spots resulting from parasecretion of estrin during pregnancy or puerperium, ophthalmalgia, dacryorrhea, withered hair, and dim lips.

Ⅷ. The Kidney Meridian of Foot-*Shaoyin*

ACUPOINTS, LOCATIONS AND INDICATIONS:

1. Yongquan (K 1): located in the center of the sole, in the depression between the 2nd and 3rd metatarso-phalangeal joint when toes are flexed.

Indications: hemicrania, hypertension, infantile fever.

2. Taixi (K 3): located in the depression between the medial malleolus and Achilles tendon.

Indications: larynagalgia, toothache, insomnia, nocturnal ejaculation, impotence, irregular menstruation.

3. Dazhong (K 4): located 0.5 cun below Taixi (K 3), at

the medial border of the Achilles tendon.

Indications: rigidity and pain of waist and spine, heel pain, asthma, hemoptysis.

4. Shuiquan (K 5): located 1 cun directly under Taixi (K 3).

Indications: irregular menstruation, dysmenorrhea, urinary incontinence, blurring of vision.

5. Zhaohai (K 6): located in the depression at the inferior border of the medial malleolus.

Indications: irregular menstruation.

6. Jiaoxin (K 8): located 2 cun above the medial malleolus, at the medial and lateral border of tibia.

Indications: irregular menstruation, diarrhea, constipation, testic edema and pain.

7. Zubin (K 9): located 5 cun directly above Taixi (K 3).

Indications: mania, hernia, pain in lower extremities.

BEAUTIFYING EFFECTS:

Improving pathologically lean constitution and hypersensitive constitution, weight loss, and regulating hypofunctions resulting from emotional discomfort, such as neurosism, facial edema, dim complexion, blurring of vision, watery stool and chronic diarrhea.

IX. The Pericardium of Hand-*Jueyin*

ACUPOINTS, LOCATIONS AND INDICATIONS:

1. Quze (P 3): located in the cubital crease at the ulnar side of the biceps brachii tendon.

Indications: soreness, pain and tremor of upper extremities.

2. Ximen (P 4): located 5 cun above the transverse crease of wrist, between tendons of palmaris longus and flexor carpi radialis muscles.

Indications: heart pain, heart palpitation, vomiting.

3. Neiguan (P 6): located 2 cun above the transverse crease of wrist, between tendons of palmaris longus and flexor carpi radialis muscle.

Indications: stomachache, vomiting, heart palpitation, amentia.

4. Daling (P 7): located in the middle of the transverse crease of wrist, between tendons of palmaris longus and flexor radialis carpi muscle.

Indications: heart pain, heart palpitation, stomachache, vomiting, epilepsy, thoraco-costal pain.

5. Laogong (P 8): located in the transverse crease in the center of the palm, between the 1st and 2nd metacarpal bones.

Indications: heart palpitation, tremor.

BEAUTIFYING EFFECTS:

Preventing and treating irritability, listlessness, and dim complexion.

Ⅹ. The Triple Energizer Meridian of Hand-*Shaoyang*

ACUPOINTS, LOCATIONS AND INDICATIONS:

1. Zhongzhu (TE 3): with clenched fist, located in the depression between the posterior borders of the capitula of the 4th and 5th metacarpal bones.

Indications: hemicrania, pain and difficulty bending and ex-

tending of palm and fingers, pain in elbow and arm.
2. Yangchi (TE 4): located in the transverse crease on the dorsum of the wrist, in the depression on the ulnar side of tendons of extensor muscles.

Indications: pain in shoulder and arm, wrist pain, malaria, diabetes.

3. Waiguan (TE 5): located 2 cun above the transverse crease on the dorsum of wrist, between ulnar and radial bones.

Indications: headache, pain and difficulty bending and extending of elbow, arm and finger.

4. Huizong (TE 7): located 3 cun above the transverse crease on the dorsum of wrist, on the radial lateral side of ulna.

Indications: deafness, epilepsy, arm pain.

5. Jianliao (TE 17): located exterior and below the acromion, in the depression 1 cun behind Jianyu (LI 15).

Indications: soreness and pain in shoulder and arm, difficulty moving shoulder joint.

BEAUTIFYING EFFECTS:

Preventing and treating furuncle, brandy nose, acne, and dermatological disorders; also effective on conjuctival congestion and eye pain, deafness and skin edema.

XI. The Gallbladder Meridian of Foot-*Shaoyang*

ACUPOINTS, LOCATIONS AND INDICATIONS:

1. Fengchi (G 20): located between the sterno-cleido-mas-

toideus muscle and the trapezius muscle, parallel with Fengfu (GV 16).

Indications: hemicrania or aching all over the head, common cold, nape rigidity.

2. Jainjing (G 21): located on midpoint of the line connecting Dazhui (GV 14) and the acromion.

Indications: nape rigidity, pain in shoulder and back, difficulty raising arm.

3. Juliao (G 29): located on midpoint of the line connecting anterior superior iliac spine and the great trochanter.

Indications: pain in waist and lower extremities, soreness and pain in sacral joint, sacro-iliilis.

4. Huantiao (G 30): located on the line connecting the the great trochanter and hiatus of sacrum, closer to the trochanter in 1/3 distance.

Indications: pain in waist and lower extremities, hemiparalysis.

5. Fengshi (G 31): located in the middle of the lateral surface of the thigh, 7 cun above the horizontal line of the popliteal transverse crease.

Indications: hemiparalysis, soreness and pain in knee joint.

6. Yanglingquan (G 34): located in the depression anterior and inferior to small head of fibula.

Indications: soreness and pain in knee joint, pain in hypochondrium.

7. Waiqiu (G 36): located 7 cun above lateral malleolus on the anterior border of fibula.

Indications: fullness in the chest and hypochondrium, pain

and flaccidity of skin, epilepsy.

8. Guangming (G 37): located 5 cun above lateral malleolus on the anterior border of fibula.

Indications: lumbago, flaccidity of lower extremities, eye pain, night blindness, mammary swelling.

9. Xuanzhong (G 39): located 3 cun above lateral malleolus on the anterior border of fibula.

Indications: headache, nape rigidity, soreness and pain in lower extremities.

10. Qiuxu (G 40): located anterior to and below lateral malleolus, in the depression on the lateral side of the tendon of muscle extensor digitorum longus.

Indications: pain in ankle joint, hypochondriac pain.

11. Zulinqi (G 41): located 1.5 cun above the end of the crease between the 4th and 5th toes on the dorsum of foot.

Indications: scrofula, hypochondriac pain, swelling and pain in back of foot, spasm in toe.

BEAUTIFYING EFFECTS:

Preventing and treating incoordination between liver and gall bladder, dyspepsia, sallow complexion and eczema.

XII. The Liver Meridian of Foot-*Jueyin*

ACUPOINTS, LOCATIONS AND INDICATIONS:

1. Taichong (Liv 3): located on the dorsum of foot in the depression between the 1st and 2nd metatarsal bones.

Indications: headache, dizziness, hypertension, infantile convulsion.

2. Ligou (Liv 5): located 5 cun above medial malleolus, in the center of the inner lateral side of tibia.

Indications: urinary incontinence, irregular menstruation, flaccidity of lower extremities.

3. Zhongdu (Liv 6): located 7 cun above medial malleolus, in the center of the inner lateral side of tibia.

Indications: abdominal pain, diarrhea, hernia, metrorrhagia and metrostaxis.

4. Zhangmen (Liv 13): located on the tip of the free end of the 11th rid.

Indications: pain in the thoraco-costal region, choking sensation in the chest.

5. Qimen (Liv 14): located directly under the nipple, in the 6th intercostal space.

Indications: pain in the thoraco-costal region.

BEAUTIFYING EFFECTS:

Removing freckles, treating depression, dysphoria and irritability caused by disorder of the liver-qi, mammary swelling and pain, mammary maldevelopment, improving dim skin, and night blindness and doltanism caused by deficiency of liver-blood.

XIII. The Conception Vessel

ACUPOINTS, LOCATIONS AND INDICATIONS:

1. Guanyuan (CV 4): located 3 cun below umbilicus.
Indications: abdominal pain, dysmenorrhea, enuresis.
2. Shimen (CV 5): located 2 cun below umbilicus.
Indications: abdominal pain, diarrhea.

3. Qihai (CV 6): located 1.5 cun below umbilicus.

Indications: abdominal pain, irregular menstruation, enuresis.

4. Shenque (CV 8): located in umbilicus.

Indications: abdominal pain, diarrhea.

5. Zhongwan (CV 12): located 4 cun above umbilicus.

Indications: stomachache, abdominal distention, vomiting, dyspepsia.

6. Jiuwei (CV 15): located below the xiphoid process, 7 cun above umbilicus.

Indications: heart and chest pain, regurgitation, epilepsy.

7. Shanzhong (CV 17): located on the front midline, parallel with the 4th intercostal space.

Indications: cough, asthma, choking sensation in chest, chest pain.

8. Tiantu (CV 22): located in the center of the supraclavicular fossa of sternum.

Indications: cough, asthma, cough with sputum.

9. Chengjiang (GV 24): located in the midpoint of the labial groove.

Indications: facial paralysis, toothache.

BEAUTIFYING EFFECTS:

Prevenging and treating abnormalities in menstruation, leukorrhea, pregnancy and delivery in females, as well as obesity, freckles and mammary maldevelopment.

Ⅳ. The Governor Vessel

ACUPOINTS, LOCATIONS AND INDICATIONS:

1. Changqiang (GV 1): located 0.5 cun below the tip of coccyx.

Indications: diarrhea, constipation, prolapse of rectum.

2. Yaoyangguan (GV 3): located under the spinous process of the 4th lumbar vertebra.

Indications: pain in waist and spine.

3. Mingmen (GV 4): located under the spinous process of the 2nd lumbar vertebra.

Indications: pain in waist and spine.

4. Shenzhu (GV 12): located under the spinous process of the 3rd thoracic vertebra.

Indications: rigidity and pain of waist and spine.

5. Dazhui (GV 14): located under the spinous process of the 7th cervical vertebra.

Indications: common cold, fever, stiffness of neck.

6. Fengfu (GV 16): located 1 cun directly above the middle of back hairline.

Indications: headache, nape rigidity.

7. Baihui (GV 20): located 7 cun directly above the middle of back hairline.

Indications: headache, dizziness, syncope, hypertension, prolapse of rectum.

8. Renzhong (GV 26): located at the junction of the upper 1/3 and lower 2/3 of the midline of the nasolabial groove.

Indications: convulsion, facial paralysis.

BEAUTIFYING EFFECTS:

Strengthening the chest and *yang*, preventing and treating

disorders in the mental, reproductive and urinary systems, and treating pathologic leanness, freckles, and dimness and roughness of skin.

XV. Extraordinary Acupoints

ACUPOINTS, LOCATIONS AND INDICATIONS:

1. Yintang (Extra): located at the midpoint on the line connecting the eyebrows.

Indications: headache, rhinitis, insomnia.

2. Taiyang (Extra): located in the depression about 1 cun behind the midpoint between the lateral end of the eyebrow and the outer canthus.

Indications: headache, common cold, eye disorders.

3. Yuyao (Extra): located in the middle of the eyebrow.

Indications: pain in the supra-orbital bone, conjunctival congestion, swelling and pain of eye, flickering eyelid.

4. Yaoyan (Extra): located in the depression 3.8 cun below and lateral to the spinous process of the 4th lumber vertebra.

Indications: lumbar sprain, soreness in waist and back.

5. Jiaji (Extra): located 0.5 cun laterally to the spinous processes from the lst thoracic vertebra to the 5th lumbar vertebra respectively.

Indications: pain and rigidity of vertebra, disorders of the viscera with health-building effects.

6. Shiqizhui (Extra): located below the spinous process of the 5th lumbar vertebra.

Indications: pain in waist and lower extremities.

7. Shixuan (Extra): located on the finger tip, 0.1 cun from the nail.

Indications: syncope.

8. Heding (Extra): located in the depression at the middle of the superior border of patella.

Indications: swelling and pain of knee joint.

9. Lanwei (Extra): located 2 cun below Zusanli (S 36).

Indications: appendicitis, abdominal pain.

10. Jianneiling (Extra): located at midpoint on the line connecting the top of anterior axillary fold and Jianyu (LI 15).

Indications: soreness and pain of shoulder joint, dyskinesia.

11. Qiaogong (Extra): located on the line between Yifeng (TE 17) behind the ear and Quepen (S 12).

Indications: headache, dizziness.

12. Dannang (Extra): located 1 cun directly below Yanglingquan (G 34).

Indications: biliary colic.

BEAUTIFYING EFFECTS:

To be introduced in the techniques of beauty massage in the following section.

Part III

The Methods and Performance of Beauty Massage

Preparations for the Performance of Beauty Massage

It is advised to perform beauty massage alone in a room, naked, without any clothes or any coverings. If it is too cold to endure, then wear clothes or apply coverings as thin as possible, so as to adapt to the "air bath" gradually. Postures should be chosen according to the different locations to be performed on, such as supine, sitting or standing. No matter which posture is assumed, the body should be relaxed, and the location to be performed on should be relaxed as fully as possible.

Breathe evenly and concentrate the mind. When you assume a posture, regulate the respiration to be even. At the beginning of the exercise, breathe into the lungs. As time passes, abdominal respiration or counter-abdominal respiration may be practiced. Meanwhile, get rid of stray thoughts and concentrate on Dantian (the location about 3 cun below the umbilicus); that is,. it is best to direct the mind toward the belly below the umbilicus; if this is impossible, one cannot force oneself to do it, still less sedulously strive for it. Coordinate respiration with will as much as possible. When inhaling, think of the word "Song" (relaxation), and when exhaling, think of the word "Jing" (tranquilization). Keep such a natural state of relaxation and tranquilization for 3 to 5 minutes. The time may be a little longer for beginners.

Make a complete preparation of massage media. Massage media should vary with seasons and symptoms, and can also be dispensed with sometimes. In spring and summer, it is hot and sweaty, so a small amount of talcum powder can be prepared to reduce the frictional resistance of the skin. In fall and winter, people with dry skin may apply a small amount of vaseline or glycerin to lubricate the skin. People suffering from headache or dizziness may use some peppermint water or cooling ointment to refresh the mind, dispel wind and relieve pain. Those suffering from joint pains due to wind-cold pathogens may apply turpentine oil. (For relevant media, see the previous part.)

The beauty media must be selected according to one's own physical conditions and actual needs; for example, some people need to eliminate acne to smarten the skin, some need to brighten the skin, some people to moisten the skin, and some need to treat dermotological diseases. Meanwhile, the selection of beauty media should be determined according to the season, weather and different applications in the morning and the afternoon. But it must be emphasized that the media must be true and effective, otherwise they will be counterproductive.

The Routine of Beauty Massage

The routine of beauty massage can be divided into two aspects: massage and practice of methods (*gongfa*).

Routine of Massage

This is divided into position, handwork and performance.

A. Positions: No matter which position is assumed, the back and the waist are required to be on the same axis.

Supine position: applicable to the head, the neck and nape, the chest and the abdomen.

Lateral recumbent position: applicable to the costal region, the waist and the buttock.

Sitting position: applicable to the entire body.

B. Handwork: It is required to be circular, soft, gentle, even, lasting, light but not floating, and heavy but not too much.

Force: from light ⟶ gradually becoming

heavy ⟶ heavy ⟶ gradually lightening.

Speed: from slow ⟶ gradually quickening ⟶ quick ⟶ gradually slowing.

Depth: from shallow ⟶ gradually deepening ⟶ deep ⟶ gradually shallowing.

Direction: To eliminate deficiency and strengthen the body, the handwork should be light and soft, countermeridianwise and clockwise, centripetal and inward, and lasting; to purge excess and remove obstruction, the handwork should be heavy, meridianwise and counterclockwise, centrifugal and outward, and the time may be shorter.

C. Performance: in a relaxed, tranquil, natural, autonomous and free state, perform the handworks on acupoints, parts or locations of disorder according to the following rules:

Shape: point ⟶ line ⟶ plane.
Order: whole ⟶ part ⟶ whole.

Method Routine

The movements should be natural and free, and will and respiration should be coordinated. Guide the movable parts of the body to do rectilinear or rotary motions.

All in all, when beauty massage is applied for

the purpose of health building and beautification, whole body massage is stressed. To prevent and treat disorders affecting beauty, there should be a coordination between local performance of massage and massage on meridians, acupoints and other locations, and practice should be conducted after. massage. Massage and practice should coordinate closely with each other. The practice of the methods should be done according to one's capability; it will be appropriate to have sensations of soreness, tingle, slight ache, and comfortable tiredness after practice. One should neither muddle through one's practice producing no sensations, nor be exhausted and overstrained resulting in self injury.

The Performance of Beauty Massage

The performance of beauty-health massage is to be as convenient and practical as possible. The handworks of massage are to be fewer and convenient, and the movements are to be convenient and easy to learn. To prevent diseases and build up health, the stress is to be laid on whole body massage; and to achieve beauty, the stress is to be laid on local performance. Meridians, acupoints and locations are to be massaged in coordination, and practice is to be done after massage. Massage and practice are to coordinate with each other closely. Massage and practice should be done according to one's capability and should vary from person to person. It will be appropriate to have comfortable and bearable sensations of soreness, tingle, pain and tiredness after the practice. One should not muddle through one's practice, with merely light sensations. Such practice will be ineffective. Nor should one be exhausted and overstrained to cause self injury. Otherwise it will affect beauty.

Common Handworks

Whether the aims of beauty and health can be attained mainly depends on the proficiency of massage handworks and their proper application. There is a large variety of massage handworks which can be roughly classified into single and compound handworks. Some handworks are similar in movements but different in names, and some are the same in names and different in movements. This chapter introduces common handworks of three types: heavy, gentle and changeable, which stimulate sensations in different ways. Special handworks will be introduced along with discussions on massage of the various parts in later sections.

1. The Handwork of Pressing

This is a changeable stimulating handwork. Use the tip of the thumb, the ventral side of the finger or the base of the palm to press the acupoints or locations, gradually increasing force to press evenly or intermittently, without changing the location of pressing. This is one of the principal handworks for beauty and health. Together with kneading and pushing, it forms the most commonly used compound handwork. It has the effects of eliminating obstruction, removing blood stasis, alleviating pain, getting rid of roughness of skin, wiping out rubella and expelling dryness and itching.

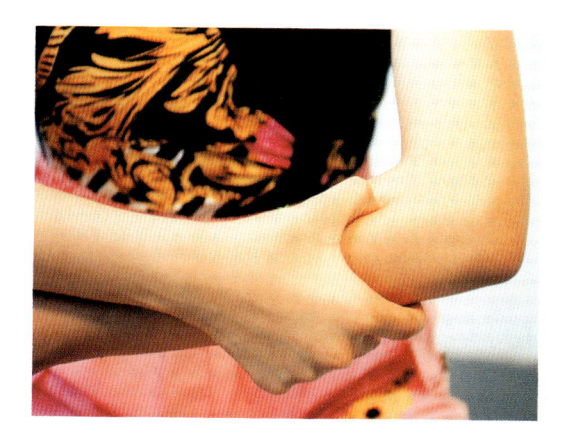

Fig. 3-1 The thumb presses (kneads) the acupoint Shousanli (LI 10).

2. The Handwork of Kneading

This is a gentle handwork of light stimulation. Put the ventral side of the finger, the base of the palm, both palms or the big or small thenar eminences on the acupoints, exert proper force and make circular kneading motions. This handwork has the effects of subduing swelling, alleviating pain, dispelling wind, removing ecchymoses, eliminating stagnancy and losing weight, and is one of the principal handworks of beauty massage.

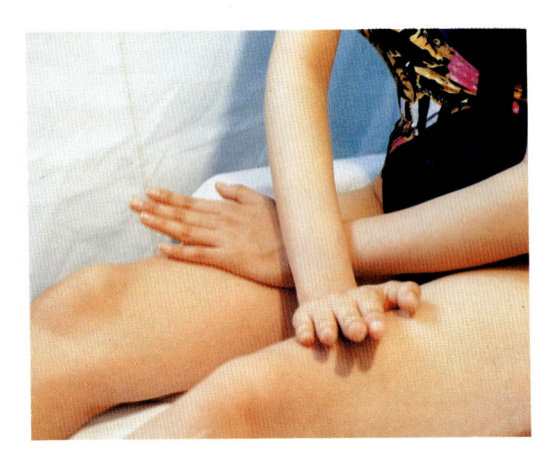

Fig. 3-2 The base of the palm kneads the inner side of the thigh.

3. The Handwork of Pushing

This is the most basic single handwork and is one of light stimulation. Pushing may be done with one finger, double fingers (dorsums of fingers or ventral sides of fingers), or the palm (big or small thenar eminences, or the base of palm). Keeping the pushing agent close to the skin, from a point to a line and to a plane simply push all the way forward; then at a small area divide into two directions, which is also referred to as wiping. Its effcets: point-shape pushing may remove blood stasis and dissolve lumps, line-shape pushing may clear and activate the meridians and collaterals, and plane-shape pushing may regulate qi and blood, dissolve lumps and remove ecchymoses, eliminate wrinkles and moisten the skin.

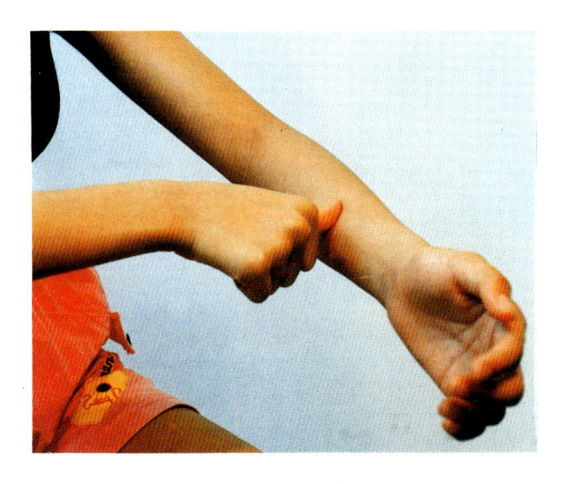

Fig. 3-3 The thumb pushes the Lung Meridian of Hand-*Taiyin*.

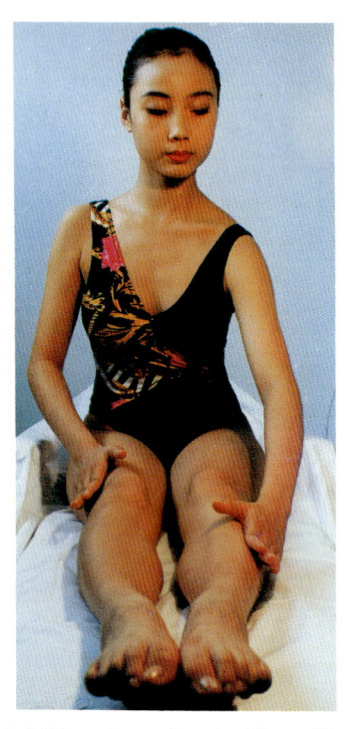

Fig. 3-4 The palm pushes the Three *Yang* Meridians of the Foot.

4. The Handwork of Punching

This is a handwork of strong stimulation and an important handwork applied to acupoints. Slightly bend the index finger, put its tip on the dorsum of the first section of the middle finger; extend the thumb, and butt its tip against the transverse crease of the first ventral section of the middle finger, with the three fingers placed one over the other. The shoulder drives the elbow and the elbow drives the wrist to punch the acupoint with the tip of the middle finger. It has the effects of removing obstruction, eliminating blood stasis, clearing meridians, getting rid of scars, and moistening and shining the skin.

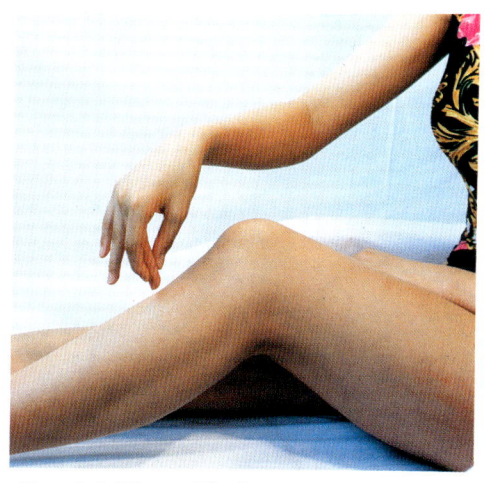

Fig. 3-5 The middle finger punches the acupoint Zusanli (S 36).

5. The Handwork of Pinching

This is a handwork of relatively strong stimulation. Use a single or both hands to form a half fist or fists. Use the thumb and the index finger or the thumb and the index, middle and ring fingers to repeatedly pinch up the skin and muscles forcefully. Its effects are similar to those of the handwork of grasping, and is applicable to people with poor constitution. Pinching is an important handwork for the beauty of the neck, the nape and the fingers.

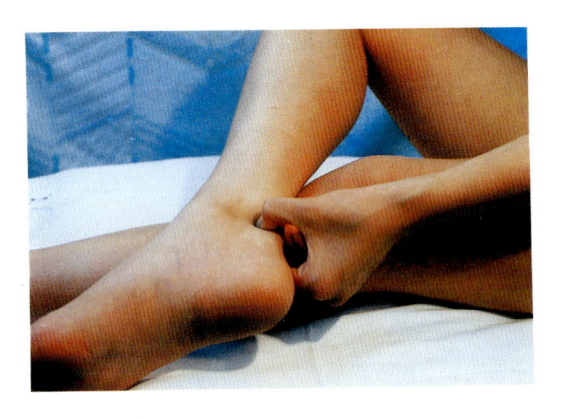

Fig. 3-6 Pinching the tendons of the heel.

6. The Handwork of Grasping

This is a handwork of relatively strong stimulation. It is similar to pinching. The force is exerted symmetrically and is so strong that it may reach the muscles and fasciae. It is usually used in combination with pinching. It has the effects of expelling wind, dispelling cold, purging heat, inducing resuscitation, dredging the meridians, regulating *qi* and blood, encouraging spirit and treating disorders affecting beauty.

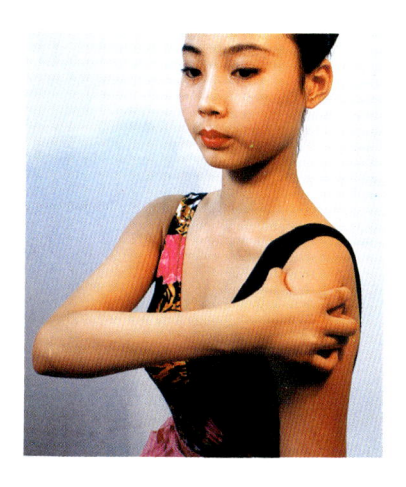

Fig. 3-7 Grasping the shoulder region.

7. The Handwork of Nipping

This is a handwork of strong stimulation. It is similar to grasping, but the force is even more concentrated. In most cases, the nail of the thumb and that of the index or middle finger are used to nip from opposite directions. Or the tips of the thumbs are used to nip a certain acupoint or location, and push and move it to both sides; this is called poking. It has the effects of inducing resuscitation, refreshing the mind, dispersing wind, alleviating pain, and treating leptochroa, rubella, dryness and itching.

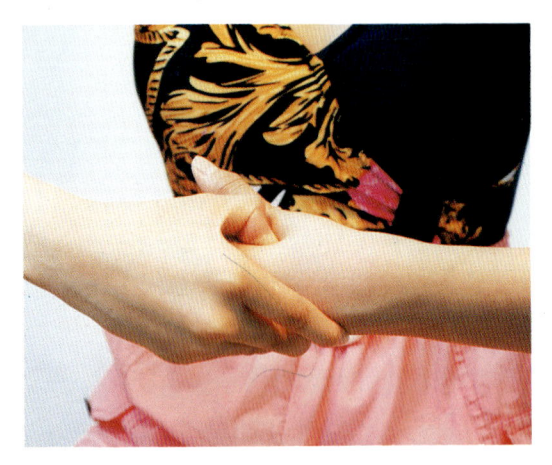

Fig. 3-8 Nipping the acupoint Hegu (LI 4).

8. The Handwork of Stroking

This is a gentle handwork of light stimulation. Put the finger tip, the whole palm, the base of the palm, or the big thenar eminence on the surface of the body, use the elbow to drive the wrist and use the wrist to drive the hand to make repeated circular motions. This handwork is mostly applied to the abdomen and the chest, and is usually coordinated with beauty media. It has the effects of regulating the flow of *qi*, regulating the stomach and spleen, activating the flow of qi, promoting blood circulation, removing ecchy-

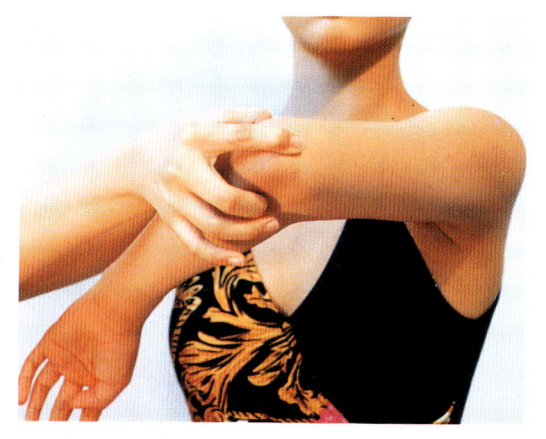

(Fig. 3-9) The middle finger pokes the acupoint Shaohai (H 3).

moses, eliminating wrinkles, and moistening and shining the skin. This is one of the principal handworks for beauty.

9. The Handwork of Rubbing

This is a warming handwork of light stimulation. Put the big and small thenar eminences or the entire palm on a location with a certain area, and rub the location to and fro rectilinearly. It is usually applied together with pushing. This is an important handwork of beauty-health massage. It has the effects of warming and dredging meridians, relieving swelling, alleviating pain, promoting the

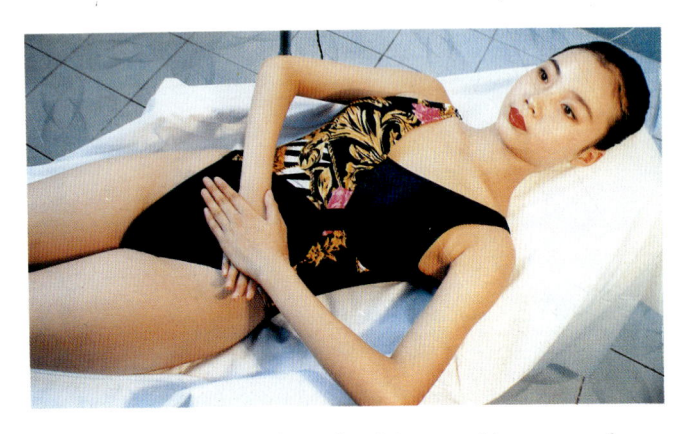

Fig. 3-10 Stroking the abdomen with superposed hands.

flow of *qi*, promoting blood circulation, eliminating scars, removing ecchymoses, and moistening the skin.

10. The Handwork of Scrubbing

This handwork is similar to rubbing. Keep the centers of the palms hollow, hold a certain location between the palms and scrub it forcefully and quickly, moving it upward, downward, to and fro at the same time. It is mainly applied to the neck, nape and lower extremities. It has the effects of regulating *qi* and blood, relaxing muscles, activating meridians, beautifying the neck

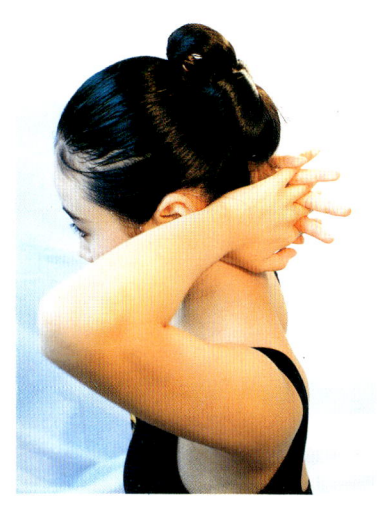

Fig. 3-11 Rubbing Fengchi (B 20) (on the nape of the neck) with palms put together.

and nape, relieving disorders of the lower extremities, and removing stasis and swelling.

11. The Handwork of Percussion

This is a stimulating handwork capable of changing from light to strong. Use the tip of finger, big and small thenar eminences, the base of palm, hollow palm or fist to percuss the affected location rhythmically and with appropriate lightness or strongness. It has the effects of improving hearing and vision, tranquilizing the mind, encouraging spirit, relaxing muscles, and increasing the elasticity of the skin.

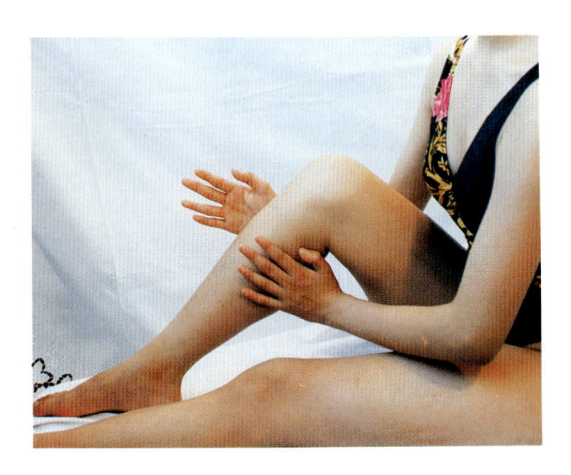

Fig 3-12 Scrubbing the shank.

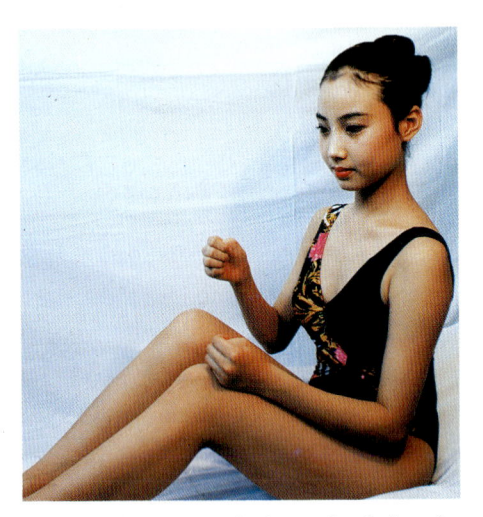

Fig. 3-13 Percussing the leg with a hollow fist.

12. The Handwork of Shaking

This is a handwork to make the joints do passive rotary motions. All the joints of the human body should make rotary motions at certain angles. The speed should be slow, the angle should vary gradually from small to big, and the force should increase gradually. Do not exert sudden force. It has the effects of easing joint movement, relieving pathologic cohesing, improving circulation and strengthening the nutrition of the tissues.

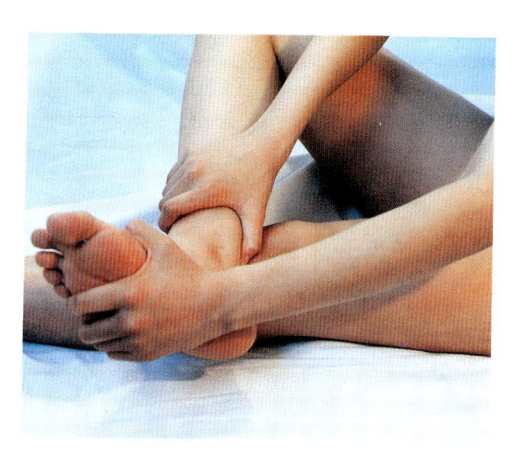

Fig. 3-14 Shaking the ankle.

Methods of Beauty Massage

According to the laws of the movement of the human body, the running orders of the meridians and the distribution of the main acupoints, start the performance from the hand, pass through the head, the neck and nape, the chest, the ribs, the waist, the leg, the foot and the abdomen, and end at the groin. The performance at each location should be conducted according to the needs of beauty, health, complexion improvement and skin moistening. Performance can be conducted emphatically at one single location. For better and lasting effects, it is advised to practice the entire set of methods according to the proper order. Each of the methods presented in the following includes three parts: the introduction mainly explains the physiological properties of the location; the procedures of performance are explained one by one according to the order of performance; and the functions are mainly the effects of the method in preventing and treating diseases; and the relevant beautifying effects are stressed at the same time.

During actual performance, it is advised to do large-area motions first, and the performance should be slow and light. Performance on acupoint locations should be rapid and heavy. In the end, increase the force gradually from small to big, and end the performance unhurriedly. The practice movements are a necessary measure to strengthen the effects, so they are also listed among the procedures of performance. Long-term persevering performance will surely lead to beauty and health. The methods are presented respectively as follows:

1. The Method to Reinforce the Heart and Make the Hand Dexterous

The hand is one of the most often moved parts of the human body and is an organ important for making a living. The hand is the starting and ending point of the three Hand *Yin* meridians and three Hand *Yang* meridians. The symptoms of the local parts of the hand usually indicate the functional states of the interior organs. Beauty massage starts from the hand, and the Method to Reinforce the Heart and Make the Hand Dexterous is the first of all the methods.

〔Procedures of Performance〕

A. Rubbing and scrubbing the hand. Put the palms together, concentrate the mind, and rub the palms forcefully till they are warm. Then rub and scrub the back of the hand alternatively, first vertically and then horizontally and circularly as if washing the hands, till the hands are rosy, moist, warm and distending. (Fig. 3-15)

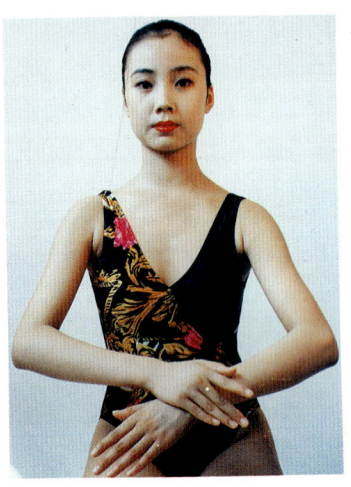

Fig. 3-15

B. Nipping and kneading the acupoints on the hand. Use the tip of the thumb of one hand to nip and knead the acupoints Taiyuan, Daling, Shenmen and inner Laogong along the inner side of the wrist of the other hand; then Yangxi, Yangchi, Yanggu, Hegu and Zhongzhu along the outer side of the wrist. Then along the finger tips and along the nail grooves, starting from acupoint Shaoshang on the thumb, according to the order of the fingers, nip and knead the acupoints Shangyang, Zhongchong, Guanchong, and Shaoze. Finally, finger by finger or with the the fingers of the two hands placed against each other, nip Shixuan forcefully.

Perform on the two hands alternatively. Nip each acupoint three to six times until it feels sore and painful. (Figs. 3-16, 3-17, 3-18)

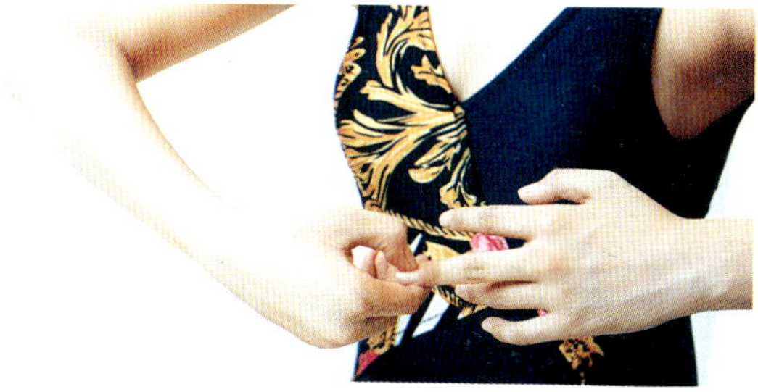

Fig. 3-16 Nipping the acupoint Zhongchong.

C. Pulling the fingers along the meridians. Employing the hand-pulling manipulation, pull each finger of both hands three times, then grasp the thumb and the other four fingers and pull them three times, to relax the finger joints. After that, employing the twisting manipulation, twist three times along the finger joints until there appear sensations of distention and numbness. (Figs. 3-19, 3-20)

D. Clenching and extending the hand. Sit-

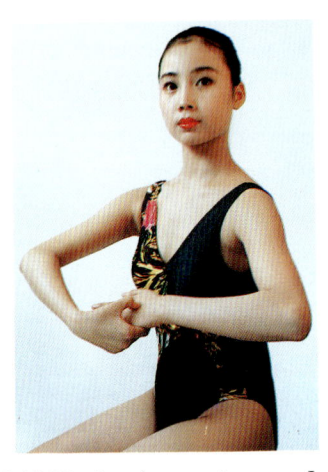

Fig. 3-17 Nipping the acupoint outer Laogong.

ting upright, tranquilize the mind, raise the hands naturally to in front of the chest and stare at the fingers. Starting from the thumb, forcefully extend the fingers in proper order; then forcefully clench them in proper order, as if counting numbers. Do each action three times. After that, extend the five fingers at the same time, stretching the palm to the maximum, and forcefully clench the fist three times. Then relax the fingers and swing and shake the wrist to end the method. (Figs. 3-21, 3-22)

〔Functions〕

It can make the fingers dexterous and the

wrist flexible, and promote the circulation of qi in the three Hand *Yin* and three Hand *Yang* meridians, regulating the qi and blood of the arms and the interior organs. At the proximal part of the hand, it can prevent and treat numbness and cold of the fingers, chilblain, tremor and pain of fingers after apoplectic paralysis, rigidity or flaccidity and senile plaque; at the distal part of the hand, it can treat common cold, vomiting, dizziness, toothache, swelling and pain of the throat, insomnia, amnesia, heart disease, scapulohumeral periarthritis and roughness and wrinkling of the skin of the hand.

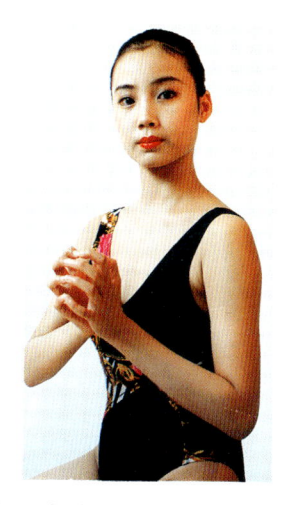

Fig. 3-18 Nipping the acupoints Shixuan.

2. The Method to Moisten the Skin and Stretch the Arms

The arms are the upper extremity of the body and connect with the shoulder and the chest. The

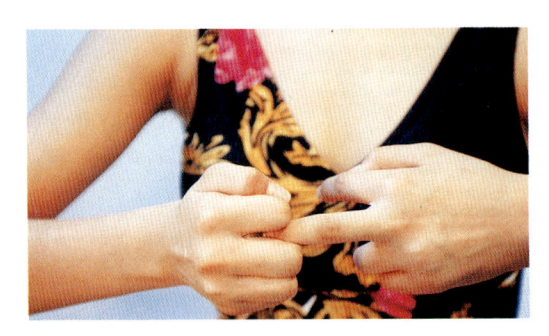

Fig. 3-19 The Handwork of Pulling Fingers.

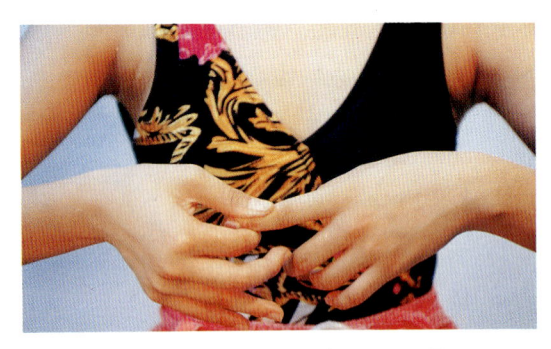

Fig. 3-20 The Handwork of Twisting Fingers.

arm has three important joints: the shoulder joint,

158

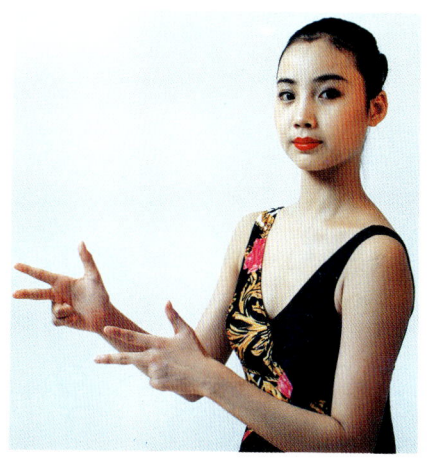

Fig. 3-21 The manipulation to extend the fingers,
the elbow joint and the wrist joint, which are the joints of the human body with the greatest scope of movement. The arm is the thoroughfare of the three Hand *Yin* and three Hand *Yang* meridians and should be unimpeded. The Maneuver to Moisten the Skin and Stretch the Arms lays stress on easing joint movement and activating meridians.

〔Procedures of Performance〕

A. Rubbing the arm. Press one palm against the inner side of the wrist of the other hand, push and rub along the inner side of the arm, namely the three Hand *Yin* meridians, to the armpit; then turn the wrist and push and rub from the

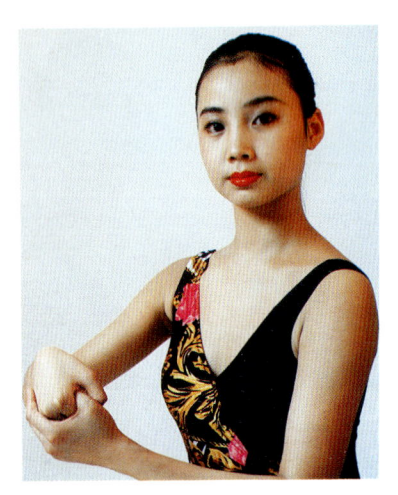

Fig. 3-22 (Taiji) The manipulation to hold the fist and swing the wrist.

shoulder along the outer side of the arm, namely the three Hand *Yang* meridians, to the back of the hand. In the light of the principle that meridianwise performance tonifies and countermeridianwise performance purges, one may do one-way or two-way rubbing several times, until there appear the sensations of warmness and distention. (Figs. 3-23, 3-24)

B. Nipping and grasping the three joints. Use the thumb, the index and middle fingers to nip and grasp the acupoints Taiyuan, Lieque, Yangchi, Daling, Shenmen, Neiguan and Waiguan at the wrist joint; Quchi, Shaohai, Xi-

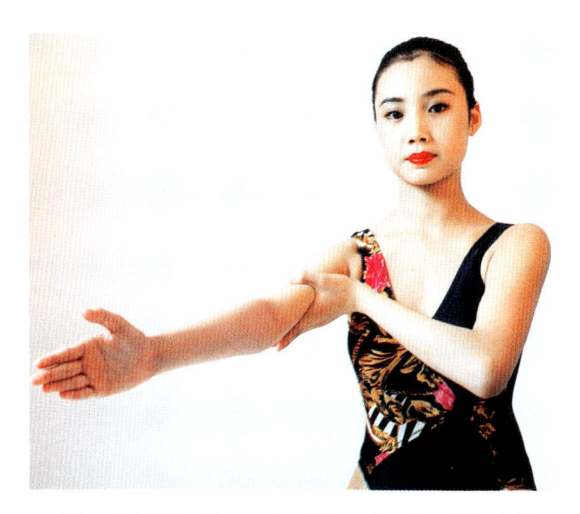

Fig. 3-23 Pushing and rubbing the three Hand *Yin* meridians.

aohai, Chize and Shousanli at the elbow joint; and Jianyu, Jianzhen, Jianliao, Jianjing, Bingfeng and Binao at the shoulder joint. Shrug the shoulder and raise the arm. This can be coordinated with the handworks of pinching, kneading, percussing and punching. Do until there appear the sensations of soreness, tingling and distention. (Figs. 3-25, 3-26, 3-27)

C. Spreading the arms. Sitting upright or standing, tranquilize the mind, be calm, relaxed and free. First cross the two hands on the two shoulders, curl up the arms and huddle up the shoulders as tightly as possible; then spread the

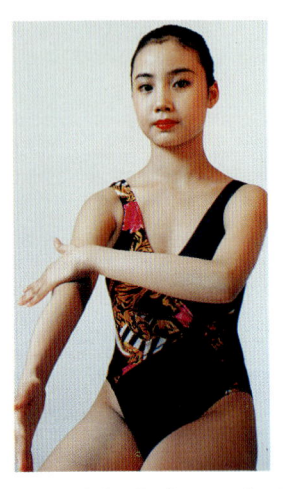

Fig. 2-24 Pushing and rubbing the three Hand *Yang* meridians.

arms and expand the chest, with the shoulder, the elbow and the wrist in a line, extend the arms forward or sideways, bend the wrists and push up the palms, with the palms not higher than the shoulders. This is the horizontal spreading of arms. Bend the elbows and wrists, and raise the hands to prop the sky; or do actions as if climbing a wall or sculling a boat; or roll up the arms and then swing the arms as if cracking whips. This is to activate the arms vertically. Bend the arms forward or backward, to activate the arms vertically. Extend the arms straight and, with the shoulders as the centers, swing the arms in big circles in both directions. This is to activate the arms rotarily. Or swing the hands as in Taiji boxing. Select one way to practice according to the needs. Pay attention to relaxation, unhurriedness and freedom.

(Figs. 3-28, 3-29, 3-30)

〔Functions〕

Locally it can prevent and treat numbness and pain of arms, paralysis of upper extremities, scapulohumeral periarthritis, tennis elbow and cervical spondylopathy; generally it can prevent and treat exopathic diseases, vomiting, stomachache, nausea, insomnia, dreami-ness, heart disease, tracheitis and hemiparalysis. It has the effects of easing joint movement, warming and dredging meridians and collaterals. It has certain beautifying and moistening effects on the skin at the shoulder, neck and arm regions, and is capable of eliminating roughness of skin, wrinkles, nevi and spots.

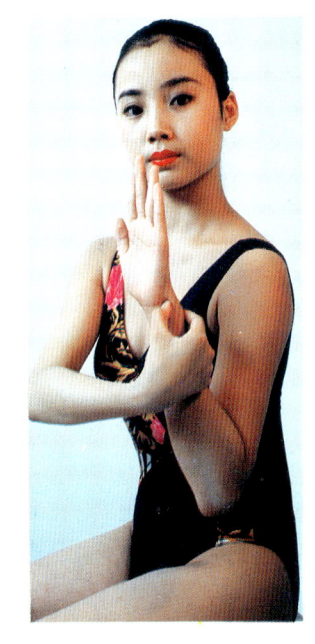

Fig. 3-25 Nipping the acupoint Shenmen.

3. The Method to Beautify the Complexion and Brighten the Eyes

The eye is the window of the liver, and the habitat for the spirit. The *Yang* meridians and collaterals mostly converge here. "The *qi* of the five *Zang* and six *Fu* organs all flushes upward into the eye to form the essence." The eye is fond of clearness and brightness and is averse to blurring and opacity. This method may promote the free flow and coordination of *qi* and blood, thus removing spiritual fatigue and strengthening vision.

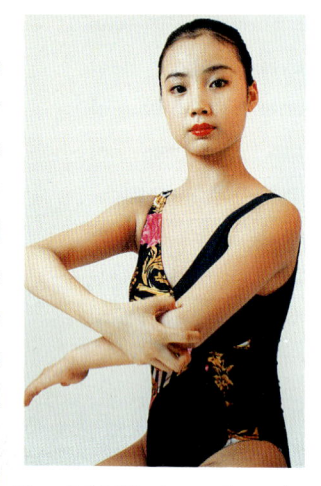

Fig. 3-26 Nipping and grasping the three acupoints at the elbow (Quchi, Shaohai and Xiaohai).

〔Procedures of Performance〕

A. Pressing and kneading the periocular region. Clenching the two hands into hollow fists, slightly bend the upper sections of the thumbs, use the raised parts of the joints to press and knead the periocular acupoints circularly. The order of the acupoints is Jingming, Zanzhu, Chengqi, Sibai, Sizhukong, Tongziliao, and Taiyang. Go from the exterior to the interior, with moderate heaviness. Do over six circles for each acupoint. Then use the ventral parts of the index and middle fingers to press and knead the eyeballs around the orbits for six circles in both directions respectively until there appear sensations of warmth and distention on the eyes. After the above movements, have a little rest with the eyes closed. (Figs. 3-31, 3-32)

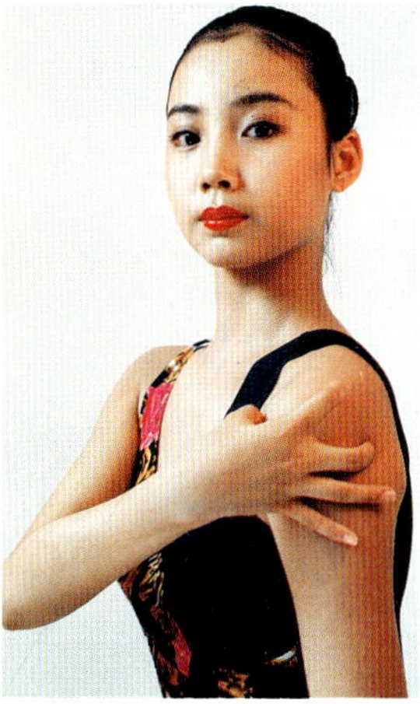

Fig. 3-27 Nipping and grasping the three acupoints at the shoulder.

B. Pinching and scraping the eyebrows and eyes. Closing both eyes, use the thumbs and index fingers to pinch the eyebrows, from Yintang to Sizhukong. Or use both hands to pinch one eyebrow at one time, until there appear sensations of soreness and distention. Then clench both hands into hollow fists, use the thumbs to press the temples; bend the index fingers into the shapes of inverted L and use the inner side of the middle sections of the fingers to scrape from Zanzhu, namely the inner superciliary end, outward to the temples; then scrape the eyeballs and the lower parts of the orbits, again from the inner parts outward to the temples. How many times may be determined according to the appearance of the sensations of warmness, distention and comfort. (Figs. 3-33, 3-34)

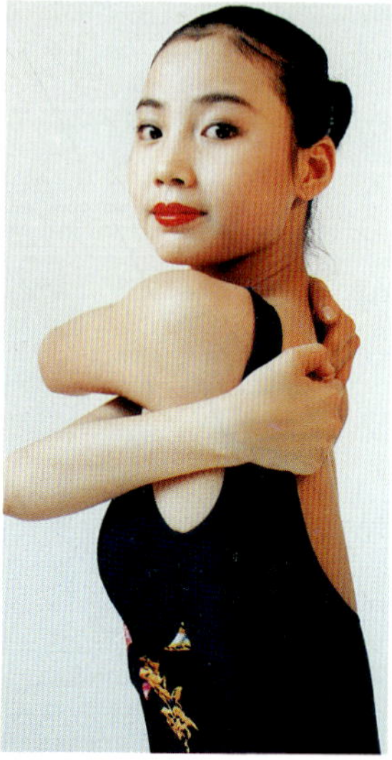

Fig. 3-28 Curling up the arms and huddling up the shoulders.

C. Four ways to exercise the eyes. Standing erect in a relaxed and tranquil state, put one palm over the other, slightly press the belly, concentrate the mind, and begin. One way is to move the eyes in six directions: open the eyes wide and

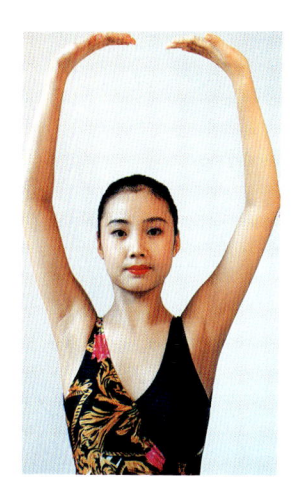

Fig. 3-29 Raising the hands to prop the sky.

look straight upward, downward, leftward and rightward, then look from downward to leftward to upward and to rightward and vice versa, circularly in both directions. Look in the six directions and cover the greatest field of vision. Make sure not to move the head and neck and perform the above action in one movement. Do six times. At the beginning it may be hard to do this automatically, in which case one may stick out a finger to direct the eyes in the six directions. The second way is to look into the distance with the eyes wide open: open the eyes to the maximum, concentrate the mind and look into the maximum distance. Concentrate the mind and gaze long and hard, paying no attention to anything else. If one feels tired, one may slowly close the eyes and then open them again to look into the distance. The third way is to rest the mind with the eyes closed: After the above two

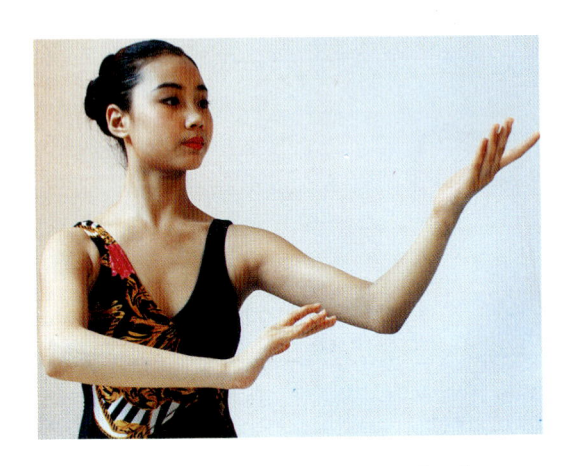

Fig. 3-30 Swinging the hands as in Taiji boxing.

ways, half-close or lightly close the eyes leaving a narrow opening, look at the tip of the nose, get rid of stray thoughts, and listen to the sound of one's own breathing or concentrate the mind on the location of Qihai (also called Dantian) in the belly. Stay this way ten minutes or so. The fourth way is to rub warm the hands, put the inner Laogongs of the palms on the eyes, lightly press and stroke the eyes six times, have a little rest and then open the eyes. (Fig. 3-35)

〔Functions〕

It can prevent and treat headache, dizziness, amblyopia, hyperopia, myopia, strabismus,

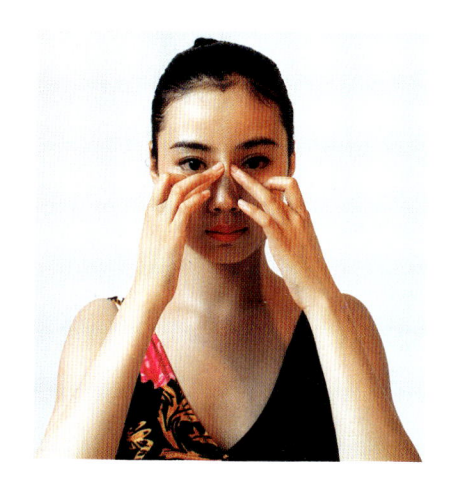

Fig. 3-31 Pressing and kneading the acupoint Jingming.

catarct, trichiasis and dark eyelids. It may prevent the occurrence of eye diseases, and has the effects of clearing away liver-fire, brightening the eyes and refreshing the spirit.

4. The Method to Induce Resuscitation and Clear Nasal Passage

The nose is a hollow passage, the window of the lung and the door of respiration. The *Yangming* meridians run into the eyes and connect with the nose. The Method to Induce Resuscitation and Clear Nasal Passage can strengthen the lung's ability to resist exopathogens and promote its dispersing

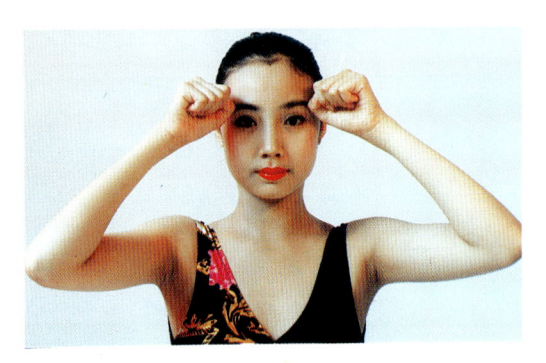

Fig. 3-32 Pressing and kneading the acupoint Sizhukong.

function.

〔Procedures of Performance〕

A. Pressing and kneading the peripheral region of the nose. Clenching one or both hands into a hollow fist(s), bend the thumb, place the raised joint(s) on acupoint Yintang above the nose, the base of the nose, acupoint Suliao above the nose, acupoints Yingxiang, acupoints Heliao on both sides and acupoint Shuigou under the nose, and press and knead circularly until there appear sensations of soreness, distention and pain. Or use the fingers to nip the acupoints. (Fig. 3-36)

B. Pushing and rubbing the nose bridge. The

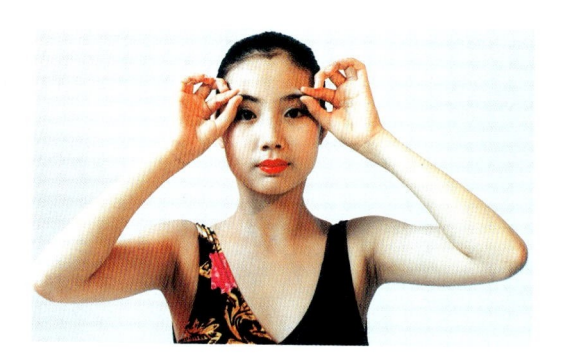

Fig. 3-33 Pinching the eyebrows.

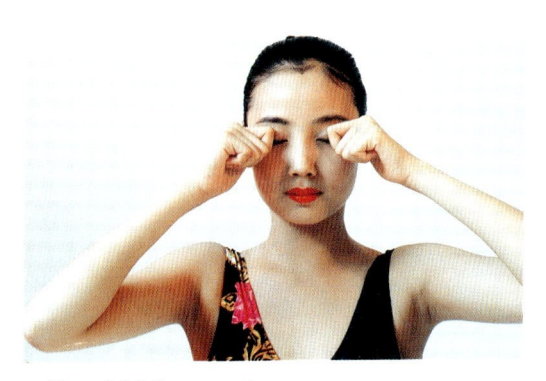

Fig. 3-34 Scraping the eyes.

hand forms are the same as in A. Put the lateral

171

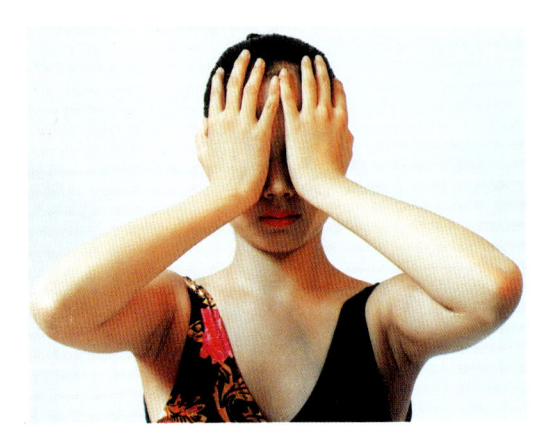

Fig. 3-35 Laogongs stroke the eyes.

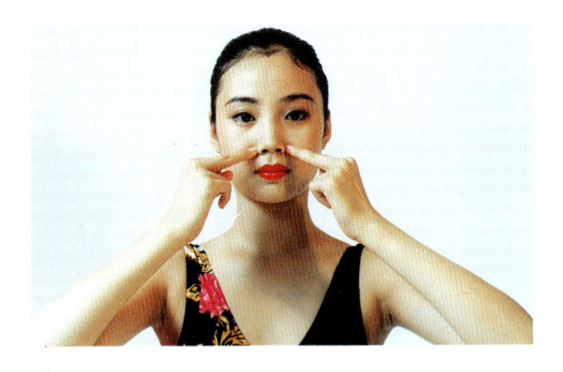

Fig. 3-36 Pressing and kneading acupoints Yingxiang.
sides of the second sections of the thumbs on the

sides of the bone of the nose bridge, forcefully and repeatedly push and rub upward to Jingming and Chengqi and downward to Yingxiang and Dicang. The two hands may push and rub in the same direction in opposite directions at the same time, until there appear the sensations of warmness and distention and the skin turns rosy. (Fig. 3-37)

C. Pinching and grasping the wings of nose. Put the tip of the index finger on the tip of the nose (acupoint Suliao), place the thumb and the middle finger on the two sides of the nose respectively, and pinch and grasp the wings of the nose. Notice to exert force in coordination with respiration and prevent suffocation. Pinch and grasp one hundred times until there appears nasal discharge. It may also be coordinated with lifting and grasping. (Fig. 3-38)

[Functions]

It can prevent and treat common cold, nasal obstruction, epistaxis, rhinorrhea with turbid discharge, anosmia, excessive discharge, atrophic rhinitis, brandy nose and facial paralysis. It has the effects of promoting osphresis, ventilating the lung and smoothing the circulation of the lung-qi.

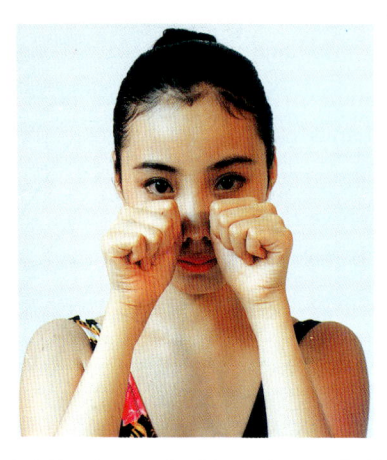

Fig. 3-37 Pushing and rubbing the nose bridge.

5. The Method to Nourish Intelligence and Improve Hearing

The ear is the window of the kidney. The *Shaoyang* meridians of the hand and the foot all converge in the ear, and the ear is closely related with the viscera. The therapeutic practice of auriculo-acupuncture shows that the physiological and pathological conditions of all the parts of the human body can be reflected in certain parts of the ear. The Method to Nourish Intelligence and Improve Hearing can not only prevent and treat local disorders but is also beneficial to the prevention and treatment of disorders of the whole organism to a

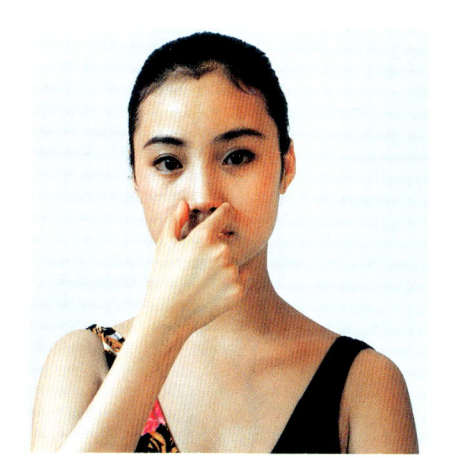

Fig. 3-38 Pinching and grasping the wings of the nose.

certain extent.

〔Procedures of Performance〕

A. Sweeping and rubbing the ears. Bend both arms inward, extend the hand naturally straight, put the palms on the ears, butt the tips of the thumbs against the earlobes, and sway the wrists to drive the palms to sweep over the ears, bringing the four fingers to rub from the front of the ears to the back of the ears; then push down the auricles and sweep and rub from the back to the front. Do this repeatedly until the ears feel warm. (Fig. 3-39)

B. Nipping the acupoints and pulling the

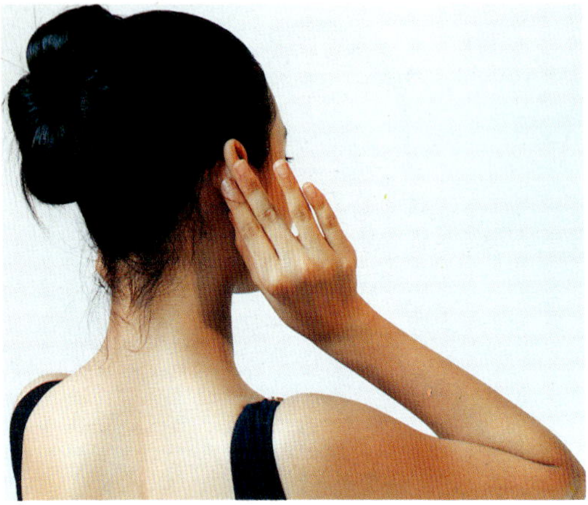

Fig. 3-39 Sweeping and rubbing the ears.

ears. Use the tips of the thumbs or the tips of other fingers to nip and knead Shuaigu and Jiaosun above the ears, Qubin, Heliao, Ermen, Tinggong and Tinghui in front of the ears, Yifeng and Yixia below the ears and Wangu and Fengchi in back of the ears, until there appear sensations of soreness, distention and pain. Then nip and knead the cavities of concha and cymba auriculae outward to the external helixes, until there is slight pain. After a little while, bend the thumbs and index fingers or the index and middle fingers into the shapes of pincers, pinch and pull the ears forward, backward, upward and downward, six

times for each direction. (Fig. 3-40)

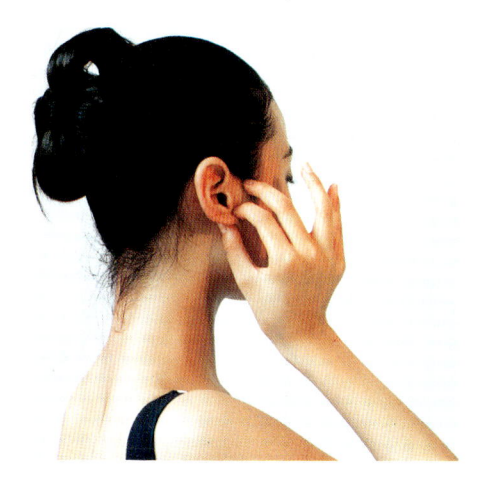

Fig. 3-40 Nipping and kneading Ermen, Tinggong and Yifeng.

C. Beating the heavenly drums: There are three ways——

a. Extend the index fingers straight, clench the other fingers into half fists with the palms facing forward, insert the two index fingers into the two earholes respectively, turn the index fingers themselves in a semicircle, repeat the turning three times, then pull out the fingers immediately, and there will be "pa", "pa" sounds in the ears. Do the action three to six times. (Fig. 3-41)

b. The palms squeezing the ears: Raise the shoulders and bend the elbows, and put the palms

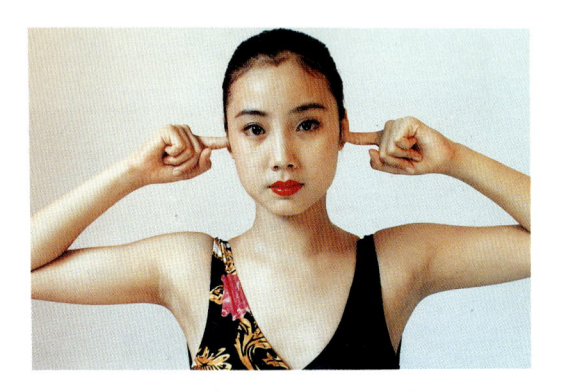

Fig. 3-41 Two fingers digging into the ears.

closely on the ears with the centers of palms over the earholes; put the tips of the middle fingers at the acupoints Fengfu and other fingers placed at the head and the neck to fix the palms. Then spread the shoulders to pull the elbows and wrists to make the palms rise and fall to press the ears. At first press slowly and forcefully, then press rapidly, producing buzzing sounds in the ears. Do the pressing thirty-odd times. (Fig. 3-42)

c. Covering the ears and percussing with the fingers: Put the palms closely on the ears with the centers of the palms facing and tightly covering the earholes. Fix the palm with the thumbs and the

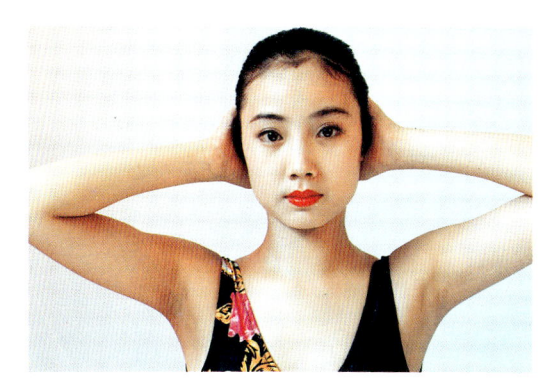

Fig. 3-42 The palms press the ears.

little fingers. Use the rest fingers, together or one by one, to percuss the occiputs of the back of the head, namely the locations of the acupoints Naohu, Fengfu and Yamen. There will be "dong, dong" sounds in the ears, like the sounds made by a beaten drum. (Fig. 3-43)

〔Functions〕

Locally it can prevent and treat deafness, tinnitus, chilblains on the ear and intra-aural disorders, strengthening hearing. Generally it can prevent and treat disorders such as common cold, rigidity of nape, dizziness, eye pain, toothache, facial paralysis and hemiparalysis. Its effects are

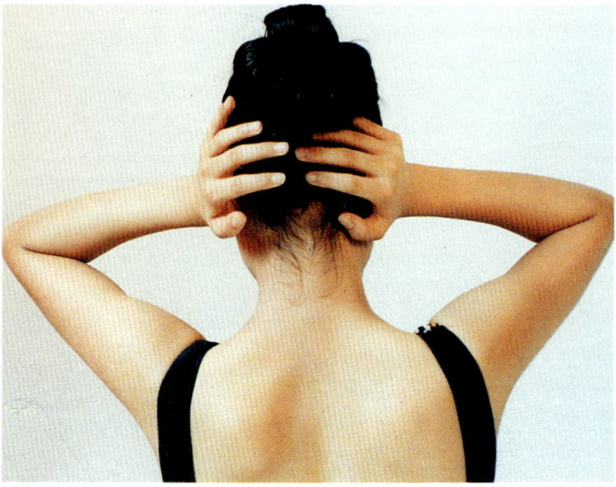

Fig. 3-43 Beating the heavenly drums.

similar to those of auriculo-acupuncture. It can regulate the functions of the organism, producing great effects with simple methods.

6. The Method to Strengthen the Mind and Beautify the Face

The head is the supreme governor of the human body. "The head is the house of intelligence." As the meeting place of all the meridians, the confluence of all *Yang* meridians, the bearer of the five sense organs and the vital dominator of life, the head is extremely important. If the head is in good health and nourishment, there will be a clear mind, surging intelligence and a healthy body. This method is the synthesis and continuation of actions such as bathing the face, combing the hair, rubbing the ears, wiping the eyes and wiping the nose.

[Procedures of Performance]

A. Pushing the forehead and combing the hair: Bend both hands naturally, put the thumbs on the temples on the two sides of the head respectively, and put the other four fingers of each hand on the eyebrows. The two hands push forcefully upward, with the fingertips slightly separated, as if combing the hair, and the thenar eminences and the bases of the palms follow the fingertips to push and rub the forehead, the crown of the head and on to the back of the head. The thumbs butt against the acupoints Fengchi, the index fingers take the lead, and the other fingers follow to push forward and gradually get together. Push and rub from the acupoint Baihui downward to Fengfu and Dazhui. One may also grasp and flick the hair to coordinate the pushing and rubbing. (Figs. 3-44, 3-45, 3-46)

B. Rubbing the ears and wiping the eyes: Follow the above step and overturn the wrists. The little fingers take the lead, the other four fin-

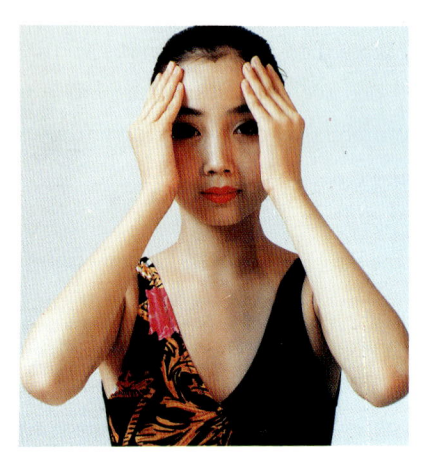

Fig. 3-44 The hands push the forehead.

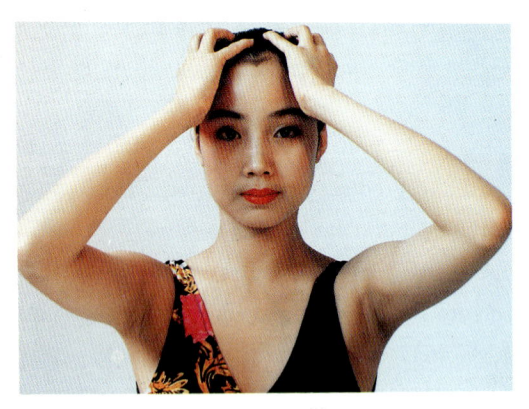

Fig. 3-45 The ten fingers comb the hair.

gers of each hand and the big thenar eminences fol-

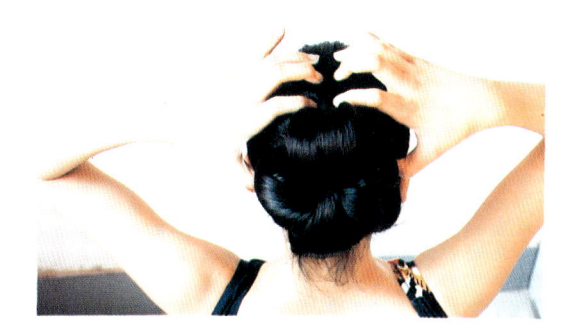

Fig. 3-46 Grasping and flicking the hair.

low to bend and rub the auricles, starting from the acupoints Fengchi, and continuing to wipe the eyeballs horizontally. The tips of the middle fingers butt against the locations of the acupoints Jingming, the ring and little fingers rest on the nose, the index fingers rest on the eyes and the thumbs press at the locations of the acupoints Quanliao. For relevant actions, see related methods in the previous part. They are omitted here.

C. Wiping the nose and bathing the face: Follow the above actions. The middle fingers exerting force and the other fingers following, rub and wipe downward along the two sides of the nose; the palms stay close to the face and rub over the mouth and lips, and end at the lower part of the mandible, like washing the face.

The order of the above actions is: From the forehead above the eyes; into the hair onto the upper part of the head; over the helix downward to the back of the head; to Dazhui; turn the wrists and rub the ears horizontally; wipe the eyes; wipe the nose downward; bathe the face; to the lower part of the mandible and put the palms together. (Fig. 3-47)

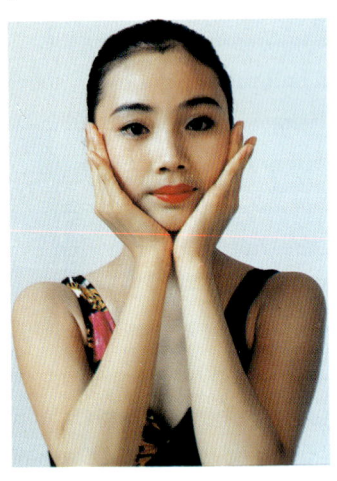

Fig. 3-47 The hands bathe the face.

Before the performance, tranquilize the mind and regulate even respiration, and be relaxed, quiet and natural. During the performance, concentrate the mind and get rid of stray thoughts. When the performance is finished, close the eyes and rest a little while.

The actions should be continuous, at a moderate speed. The actions may be done several or dozens of time according to one's physical condition. They can be coordinated with smearing one's own saliva.

D. Nipping and kneading the major acupoints: Use one, two, three or even four and five fingers to nip and knead the acupoints at the same time or use the ten fingers to percuss and punch the acupoints on the head. The often used acupoints on the forehead are Taiyang, Yintang and Yangbai; the often used acupoints on the head are Shenting, Shangxing, Baihui, Touwei, Tianchong, Naohu, Yuzhen, Fengfu and Fengchi; and the often used acupoints on the face are Xiaguan, Ermen, Yifeng, Tongziliao, Quanliao, Jingning, Yingxiang, Renzhong and Chengjiang. (Figs. 3-48, 3-49, 3-50, 3-51, 3-52, 3-53, 3-54)

〔Functions〕

Locally it can prevent and treat aching all over the head, hemicrania, listlessness, dizziness,

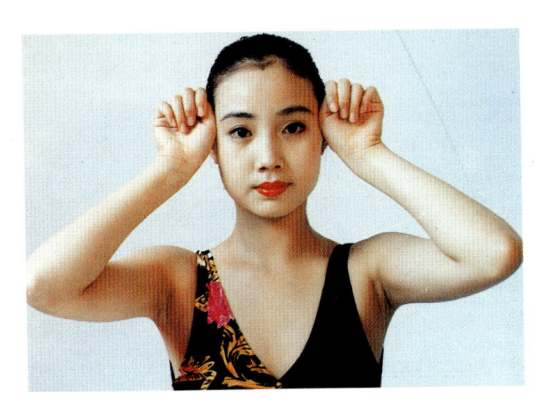

Fig. 3-48 Kneading Taiyang.

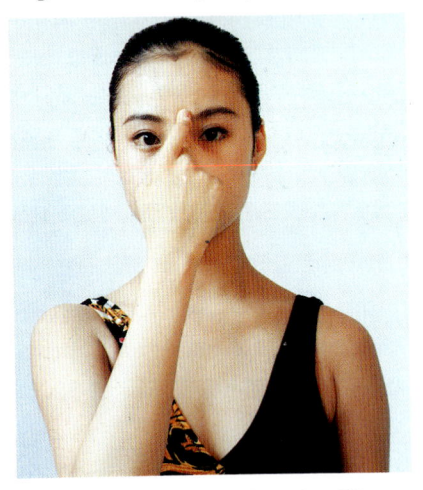

Fig. 3-49 Pressing and kneading Yintang.

dreaminess, insomnia, baldness, poliosis, tinni-

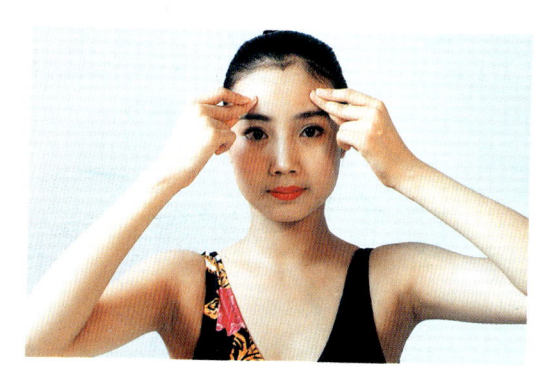

Fig. 3-50 Kneading Yangbai.

tus, nasal obstruction, blurred vision; also facial spots, nevi, wrinkles and acne. Generally it can prevent paralysis and numbness of extremities, deafness, aphasia, hypertension and facial paralysis. It has the effects of tonifying the brain, refreshing the mind and beautifying the face.

7. The Intraoral Method for Longevity

The mouth is one of the important sprouts and openings of the human body. The mouth and lips are governde by the lungs and are the superficial windows of the lungs. The teeth and the tongue in the mouth are particularly important. The teeth

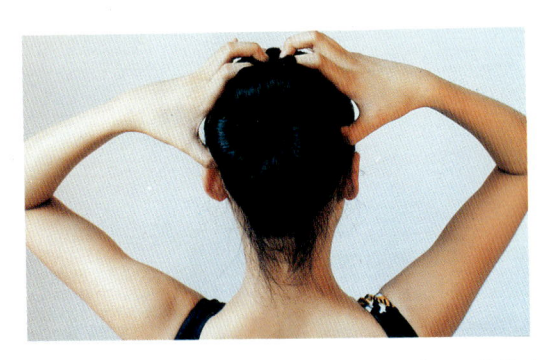

Fig. 3-51 Nipping and kneading Yuzhen, Baihui, Shangxing and Shenting.

are the terminals of the bone, pertain to the kidney and connect with the *Yangming* meridians of the hand and foot. The tongue is the sprout of the liver, and connects with the liver and spleen meridians. The saliva in the mouth moistens the five interior organs. Only when the teeth and tongue are strong and healthy and the saliva is sufficient can they benefit digestion, promote voice, boost spirit and beautify complexion. This method is divided into three submethods: to solidify the teeth, to strengthen the tongue, and to swallow saliva. They are introduced respectively in the following.

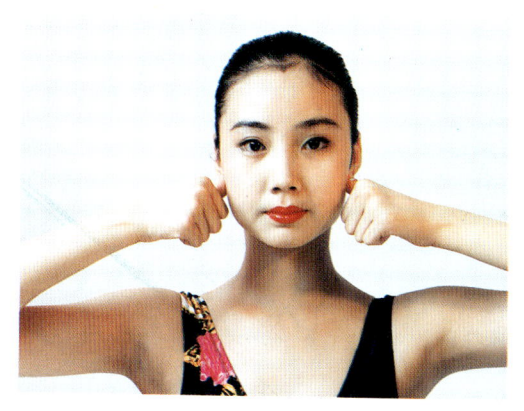

Fig. 3-52 The thumbs press and knead Xiaguan.

〔Procedures of Performance〕

A. The method to solidify the teeth. It can be done in three ways.

a. Closing the mouth and gritting the teeth. Keep the body erect and relaxed, tranquilize the mind and close the mouth. Keep the upper and lower teeth close to each other without separation. Grit forcefully, from the posterior teeth gradually to the incisor teeth. Exert force on one side or on both sides at the same time, until the cheeks feel sore and distending and the saliva increases greatly.

b. Closing the mouth and knocking the teeth. The position of the body is the same as

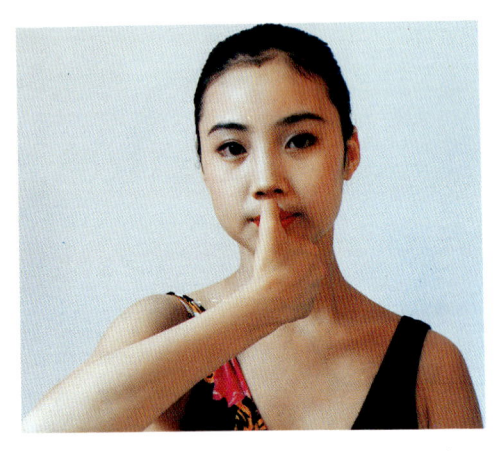

Fig. 3-53 The thumb nips and kneads Renzhong.

above. Lightly close the mouth, keep the upper and lower teeth exactly against or staggered with each other, and knock the teeth rhythmically producing a chattering sound, from slowly to quickly and from lightly to heavily, until the teeth feel tingling and distending and there appears saliva in the mouth. (Fig. 3-55)

c. Pressing and kneading the gums. Wash the fingers and put them into the mouth, and press and knead the gums, with the index fingers taking the lead, until the gums have sore and distending sensations. (Fig. 3-56)

B. Strengthening the tongue. There are two

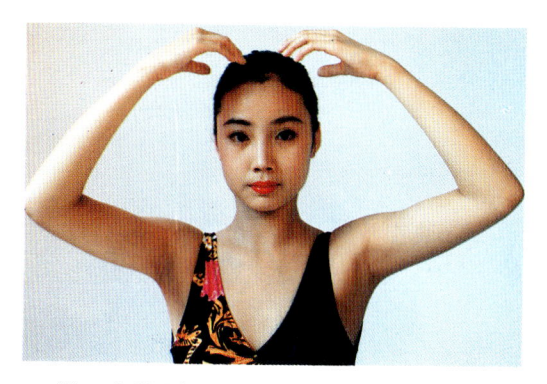

Fig. 3-54 The ten fingers percuss and punch the acupoints.

ways.

a. Stirring the tongue. Tranquilize the mind and relax the body, then lightly close the mouth. The tongue touches the inner and outer gums to make repeated circular licking motions, as if stirring something (so it is also referred to as "the red dragon stirs the sea"), until the tongue feels tingling, the cheeks feel distending and there is a mouthful of saliva.

b. The static tongue butting against the palate. In ordinary silent time, tranquilize the mind, relax the cheeks, close the mouth and butt the tongue against the upper palate. It is better if

191

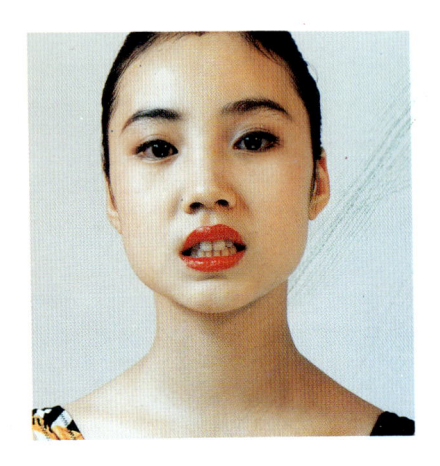

Fig. 3-55 Knocking the teeth.

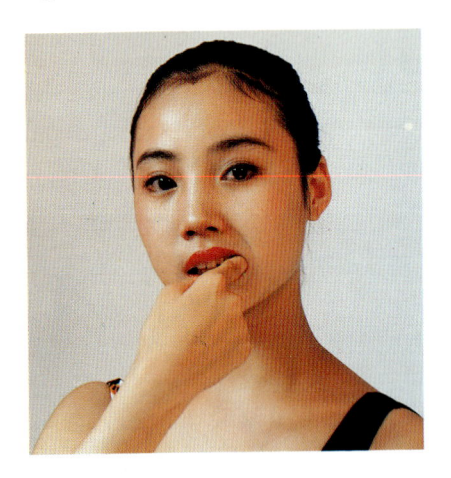

Fig. 3-56 Pressing and kneading the gums, you concentrate the mind on Dantian.

c. Swallowing the saliva. Close the mouth, grit the teeth, bulge the cheek and stir the tongue as if rinsing the mouth; this makes saliva flow autonomously in the mouth. When saliva fills the mouth, swallow it forcefully three times or more. Note: swallow it with a gurgling sound and think about sending it into the belly. (Fig. 3-57)

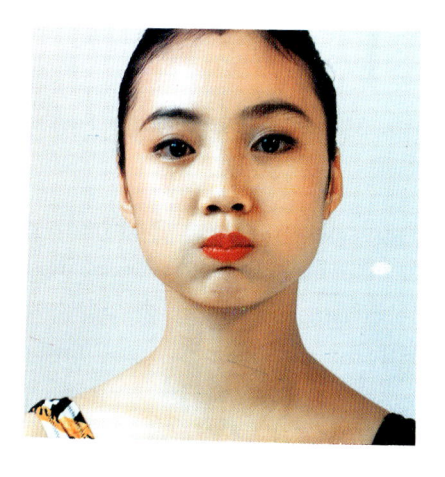

Fig. 3-57 Stirring the tongue and swallowing the saliva.

〔Functions〕

It can prevent and treat swelling and pain of the teeth, odontoseisis, odontoptosis, gingival bleeding, gingival atrophy, gingival swelling and pain, sausarism aptyalia, wry tongue, glossolysis, tongue ulcer, dizziness, vexation and dry stool. It may enhance chewing ability and strengthen digestive function. Long-term exercise of this method may subdue the pathogenic fire of the five *zang* organs and regulate the *qi* and blood of the four extremities. It has the effects of refreshing the mind and relieving dryness, as well as detoxication and immunization. It is a very effective method for beauty, health and longevity.

8. The Method to Beautify the Face and Relax the Neck

The neck supports the head upward, connects the chest, the back and the viscera downward, joins the shoulders and arms at the sides, and contains the throat and other passages inward. The Conception Vessel runs over the front of the neck, the Governor Vessel runs over the back of the neck, and the three *Yang* meridians of the hand and foot run over the two sides of the neck. As an important pass for respiration and food, the neck should be unimpeded and should not be obstructed. This method may relax the neck and promote passage in the throat.

[Procedures of Performance]

A. Kneading and grasping the front of the

neck. Clench one hand into a hollow fist, place the index finger horizontally on the acupoint Chengjiang below the lower lip, and use the tip of the thumb to knead the acupoint Lianquan. Bend the middle finger of the other hand lightly into a hook and knead the acupoint Tiantu. The two hands may perform at the same time, until there appear sensations of numbness and distention. Then use one hand along the two sides of the neck, especially the throat, along the several meridians, from inside to outside and form upward to downward knead and grasp the acupoints Renying, Yongtu, Qishe, Futu, and Tianding. Finally use the two hands to stroke, rub, pinch and lift the neck from outside to inside and from back to front alternatively, until there appear sensations of warmness and distention. (Figs. 3-58, 3-59)

B. Pressing and rubbing the back of the neck. Raise the shoulder and bend the elbow. The middle finger exerts force and the other fingers coordinate and follow to press along the spinous processes of the cervical vertebrae from the acupoint Fengfu down to the acupoint Dazhui; then with the ten fingers of the two hands cross with each other, the bases of the two palms stationed at the acupoints Fengchi on the two sides respective-

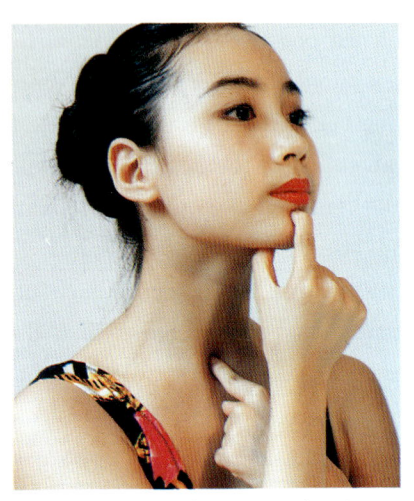

Fig. 3-58 The two hands nip the three acupoints (Chengjiang, Lianquan and Tiantu).

ly, press and rub forcefully, until there appears warmness. For this action, one may refer to the handwork of rubbing. In addition, one may press and knead the acupoints Dazhui and Fengfu with one hand, and pinch and grasp the acupoints Tianrong, Futu and Renying on the two front sides of the neck with the other. (Fig. 3-60)

C. Relaxing the neck in six directions. This is a method to exercise the neck region. Stand erect, regulate breath, and relax the neck. Extend the head forward, backawrd, leftward and rightward to the maximum, then make clockwise and counterclockwise rotations. Note theat the

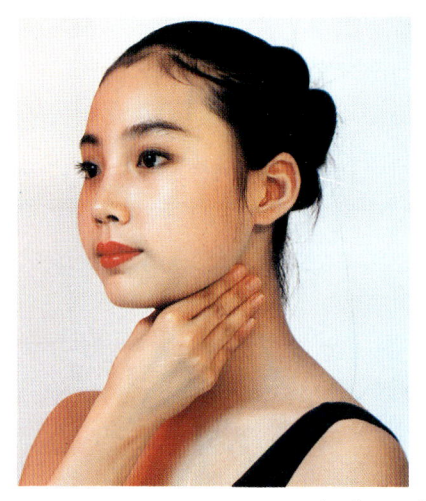

Fig. 3-59 Kneading and grasping the front of the neck.

motions in the six directions should be slow, the neck should be relaxed, and not to hold breath or extend the head rigidly.

〔Functions〕

It may prevent and treat sore and swollen throat, asthma, hiccup, cough, vomiting, hoarseness, slurred speech, rigidity of neck, wrinkling and ptosis of the skin of the neck, cervical disorders, and headache, dizziness and numbness of extremities caused by cervical disorders. It has the effects of clearing obstrctions of the throat, relaxing the neck, promoting the circulation of qi and relieving spasms.

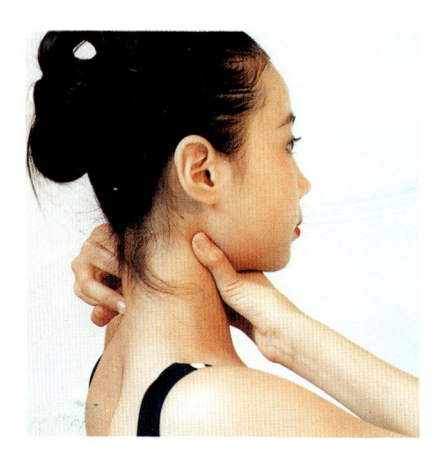

Fig. 3-60 The two hands relax the neck.

9. The Method to Expand the Chest and Costa (Appended with the Method to Plump the Breasts)

The chest houses the liver and the lung and is the base for blood generation and respiration. It should be broad and wide. The costa shelters the liver and the spleen, and the *Jueyin* and *Shaoyang* meridians of the foot run along the two costal regions and the axillary fossae. The chest and costa connect with the neck in the upper part and join the abdomen and waist in the lower part, influencing the throat and acting on the stomach and intestines. They should be spacious and unobstructed.

[Procedures of Performance]

A. Pushing and rubbing the clavicular fossa: Put the thumb at the location of the acupoint Tiantu, bring the middle and index fingers together and extend them straight, and exert force mainly with the ventral part of the middle finger to push and rub the clavicular fossa repeatedly. Alternate the two hands to push and rub the clavicular fossa on the opposite side respectively, until there appear distention and pain. (Fig. 3-61)

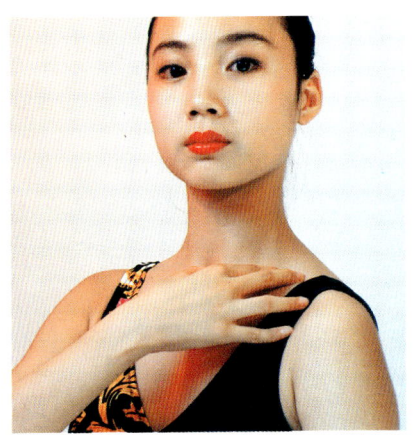

Fig. 3-61 One hand pushes and rubs two acupoints (Tiantu and Quepen)

B. Pressing and kneading important acupoints. Use the fingers or the thenar eminences, both or separately, to press and knead the acupoints Yunmen, Qihu, Huagai, Yingchuang, Xiongxiang, Shanzhong, Jiuwei, Qimen and Zhangmen, especially Shanzhong. (Fig. 3-62)

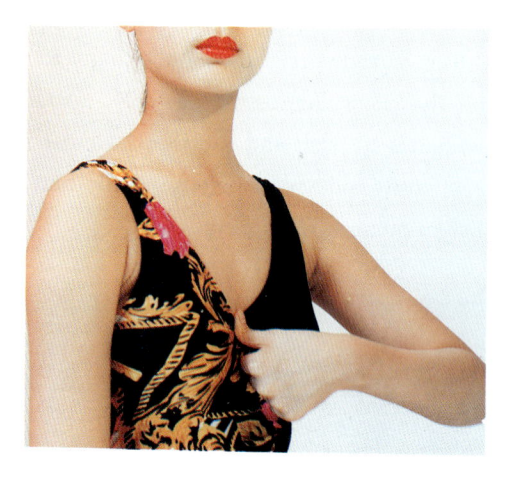

Fig. 3-62 The thumb presses and kneads Shanzhong.

C. Rubbing and bathing in three directions. Both hands bend naturally into hooks, and the fingers exert force to rub and wipe from the chest to the abdomen from the upside to the downside, vertically and rectilineally. Then rub and wipe from the left to the right and from the right to the left, horizontally and rectilineally. After that, rub and wipe along the sternocostal space from the inside to the outside, curvingly and obliquely. Do each action six times, then change to using the palms to rub and wipe as above. Note not to hold breath during the performance. It may also be coordinated by percussing the sternocostal region with the fingers, palms or fists, but the percussion should be light and slow. Heavy and rapid percussion is prohibited. (Fig. 3-63)

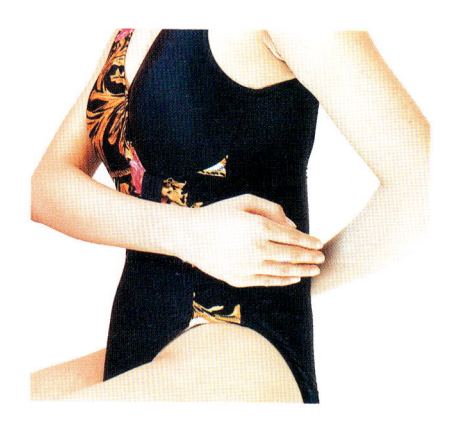

Fig. 3-63 The palm percusses the costal region.

D. Spreading the arms and expanding the chest. Frequently spread the arms and expand the chest to coordinate with the above actions. Raise the arms upward, spread the arms outward and swing the arms backward, coordinating with rhythmical respiration, to stengthen the exercise of the chest, enhance pneumocardial functions and increase the beauty of the lines of the human body.

[Functions]

It can prevent and treat disorders such as chest distress, chest pain, cough, asthma, sternocostal fullness, incoordination between the liver and the spleen, heart disease, trachietis and chronic hepatitis. It has the effects of facilitating the flow of the lung-qi to relieve asthma, relieving stuffiness of the chest and regulating the flow of qi, tonifying the heart and relieving spasms, soothing the liver and strengthening the spleen.

[Appendix] The Method to Plump the Breasts

The breasts of the female are of great value in her beauty and directly influence the curvilinear beauty of the figure. The plumpness and prominence of the breasts are the important indexes of the health and beauty of the female. The studies of scholars both at home and abroad show that massage is an effective way to plump the breasts.

[Procedures of Performance]

A. Pushing and rubbing the breasts. Lightly spreading the fingers of both hands, use the ventral parts of the fingers to push and rub radially from the nipples outward. Gradually separate the fingers broadly, and alternate the two hands in the performance (the left hand performs on the right breast and the right hand performs on the left breast). Do 20 times.

B. Propping and kneading the breasts. The left hand props up the right breast, lightly presses and kneads it from the outside to the inside, and gradually pushes it from the downside to the upside, about 3 circles and 60 times. The right hand performs on the left breast in the same way. (Fig. 3-64)

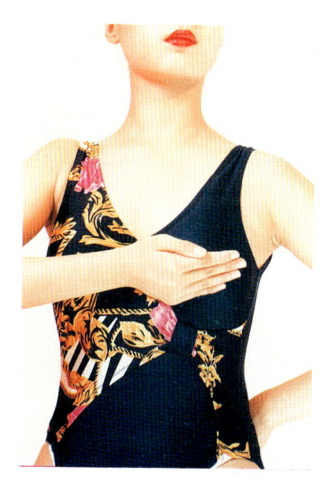

Fig. 3-64 Propping and kneading the breast.

C. Grasping and wiping the breasts. Separate the fingers of both hands, and place them around the breast on the same side respectively. First use the fingers to knead the peripheral regions of the breasts, then place the centers of the palms over the nipples, gradually draw the fingers together and grasp and wipe the breasts to the nipples. If the nipples are depressed, they might be pulled out properly. Usually do 30 times. (Fig. 3-65)

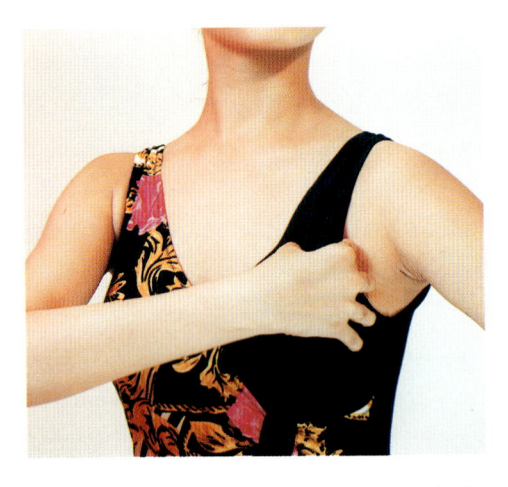

Fig. 3-65 Grasping and wiping to plump the breasts.

D. Pressing and kneading important acupoints. Use the fingers to press and knead the acupoints Quepen, Xiongxiang, Shanzhong, Rugen and Huagai, and press and knead from the downside to the upside along the direction of the sternocleidomastoid muscles to the acupoints Quepen and Jianjing. 20 times for each acupoint.

〔Functions〕

It may treat mammary maldevelopment,

crater nipples, small breasts and mastoptosis. It has the effects of increasing estrogen, promoting mammary development and promoting the functions of the mammary glands.

10. The Method to Strengthen the Waist and Tonify the Kidney

The waist is the location of the kidney. Most meridians of the body pass through the waist, and the Belt Vessel runs around the waist like a belt. The waist moves under the weight of the body, so its symptoms are mostly heaviness and pain; though they are not complicated, they are widely involved. If the waist is diseased, the whole body will be uneasy, which is why people say the waist is important. Inside the waist stays the kidney. The kidney is the origin of congenital constitution and is liable to be insufficient. It is fond of warmth and is averse to cold, so it likes to be warmed and tonified.

[Procedures of Performance]

A. Rubbing and scrubbing the sides of the waist. Put the palms or fists on the two sides of the waist, with the acupoints Shenshu at their centers; rub and scrub to and fro repeatedly upward to under the the the twelve ribs and downward to the buttocks and the iliac region, until there appear warmth and perspiration. It may also be coordinated with the handworks of pressing and kneading. The above is the sitting performance. When lying on one side, one may perform on the other side with one hand. (Fig. 3-66)

B. Percussing and patting the lumbosacral portions. Bend the arms behind the back, and use the backs of the fists or the bases of the palms to percuss or pat along the lumbar and sacral vertebrae up and down alternatively several times, until there appear numbness, distention and soreness. (Fig. 3-67)

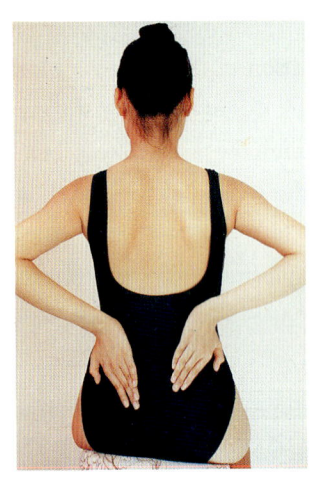

Fig. 3-66 Rubbing and scrubbing the sides of the waist.

C. Pushing and grasping the Governor Vessel. Ask other people for help to push and press the Governor Vessel from the acupoint Dazhui to Changqiang and the portions on the two close sides of the spinal column. Pinch and grasp six times re-

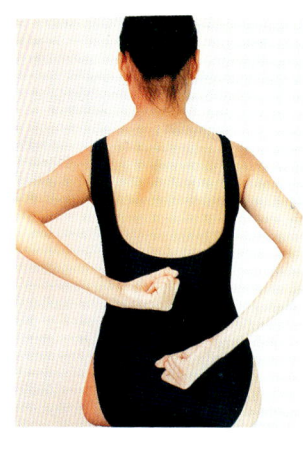

Fig. 3-67 The fists percuss the lumbosacral portion.

spectively. (Figs. 3-68, 3-69)

D. Moving the waist in six directions. Sitting upright, tranquilize the mind and regulate respiration. Bend forward, backward, leftward and rightward, and sway the waist circularly clockwise and coun-

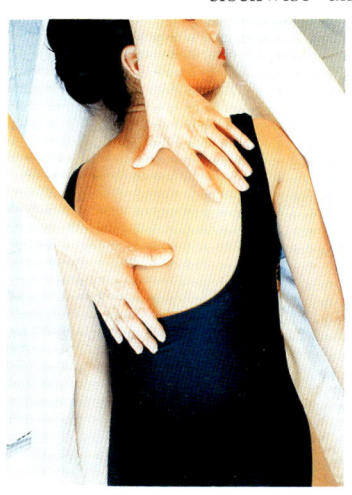

Fig. 3-68 Pressing and pushing the Governor Vessel.

207

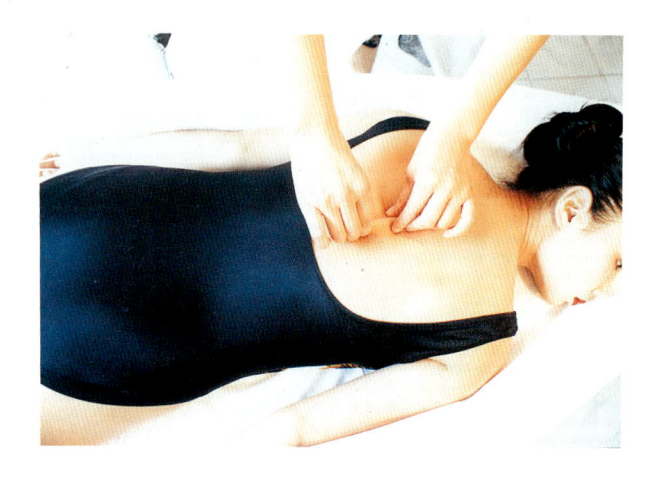

Fig. 3-69 Pinching and grasping the Governor Vessel.

terclockwise. Keep the legs and buttocks fixed and unmoving. Breathe rhythmically and relax the body. The range should be large while the speed should be slow. The times of the motions are to be determined by the need.

[Functions]

Long time exercise of this method may prevent and treat lumbago, lassitude in legs, sprain of waist, lumbar muscle strain, atrophy of waist muscle, sciatica, hyperosteogeny, protrusion of intervertebral disc, nocturnal ejaculation, impotence, premature ejaculation, nephritis, prostatitis, neurosism, dark eyelids, latent sores, disorders caused by nephroptosis that affect beauty and irregular menstruation. It has the effects of expelling wind and dampness, strengthening the waist and kidney, nourishing the essence, warming the waist and tonifying the kidney.

11. The Method to Strengthen the Leg

The leg is an important limb to support the body and has three major joints: hip, knee and ankle. The leg is mostly governed by the spleen, and the six foot meridians run along it. Commonly seen are muscular and joint pains and dyskinesia, caused by the invasion of pathogenic wind, cold and dampness. The health of the leg is beneficial to the waist. To strengthen the leg may expel many diseases. The acupoint Zusanli which is called the "longevity point" may, if massaged constantly, not only treat leg disorders but also reinforce the spleen and stomach and strengthen the body. Persevering exercise of the legs method may make the steps nimble and the activities agile. There are many ways to exercise the legs. In addition to various standing stances, there are also various kinds of kicking and walking methods which are not discussed here.

[Procedures of Performance]

A. Punching and grasping the important acupoints on the foot meridians. Assume the sitting position and relax the body. Use the middle fingers of both hands at the same time to punch or grasp the acupoints one by one, starting from the groin above the leg of the same side, from the upside to the downside and from the inside to the outside. Perform six times for each acupoint, and decide the heaviness yourself. Along the meridians of Foot-*Yangming*, the acupoints Biguan, Yinshi, Zusanli, Fenglong and Jiexi may be selected. Along the meridians of Foot-*Shaoyang*, the acupoints Huantiao, Fengshi, Yanglingquan, Guangming and Qiuxu may be selected. Then use the right hand to perform on the lateral side of the left leg and the left hand to perform on the lateral side of the right leg, selecting Qimen, Xuehai, Yinlingquan and Sanyinjiao along the meridians of Foot-*Taiyin*, Wuli, Yinbao, Ququan and Xiguan along the meridians of Foot-*Jueyin*, and Yingu, Zubin and Fuliu along the meridians of Foot-*Shaoyin*. For grasping, just select Chengfu, Yinmen, Weizhong, Chengjin, Chengshan and Kunlun along the meridians of Foot-*Taiyang*. Note to regulate the postures and positions of the legs for grasping. (Fig. 3-70)

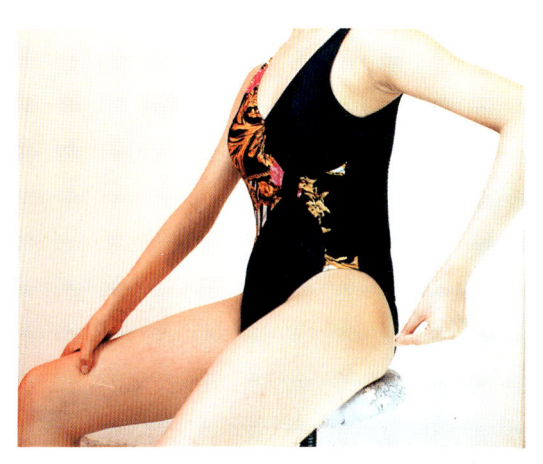

Fig. 3-70 Punching and grasping the important acupoints (punching Huantiao and grasping Xuehai).

B. Clasping and rubbing the legs. Place one hand under the ilium on the outer side of the base of one thigh, place another hand on the groin, with the fingertips pointing at each other, and clasp one leg with both hands. First scrub forcefully, then rub downward to the ankle. After that, forcefully scrub and rub backward to the base of the thigh repatedly, until there appear warmness and distention. One may also perform on the thigh and shank separately. (Fig. 3-71)

C. Nipping and kneading the knees. Assume the sitting position, with the legs stretched straight or bent naturally. Press both hands on the

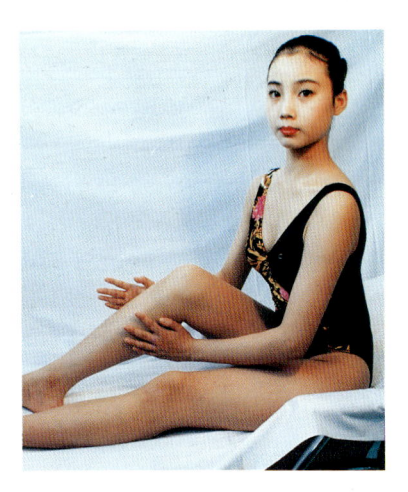

Fig. 3-71 Scrubbing and rubbing the legs.

knees, point the bases of the palms at the acupoints Heding, bend the five fingers lightly like hooks, and place the fingers at the peripheral regions of the knees with the index and ring fingers placed on the two lateral sides of the knees respectively. Suspend the elbow and swing the wrists, and exert force with the fingertips to nip and knead along with the swinging, until there appear warmness, soreness and distention. (Fig. 3-72)

D. Nipping and lifting the Achilles tendons. Assume the sitting position. Bend one leg and place it on another leg, or bend both legs, with the toetips touching the ground and the heels

212

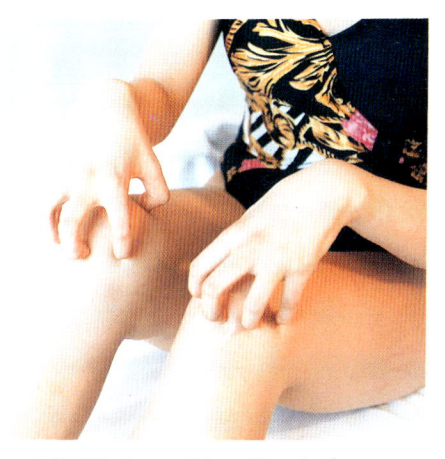

Fig. 3-72 Nipping and kneading the knees.

pointing upward. Use one or both hands to nip and lift the Achilles tendons of both heels along the lower sections of the shanks to the end of the heels, until there appear soreness and pain. For this action, refer to the handwork of nipping.

E. Shaking the ankles and pulling the toes. Assume the sitting position. Bend one leg into the shape of the number "4" and place it on the other leg. Use one hand to hold the knee of the bent leg, holding the center of the palm of the other hand over the center of the foot, grasp the five toes of the foot and bend, pull and stretch them upward, downward, leftward and rightward, and turn them circularly clockwise and counterclockwise, six times in each direction. Then bend the index and middle fingers like pincers, and pinch, nip, pull, stretch and comb the five toes, six times each. For this action, refer to the handwork of shaking.

F. Activate the three joints of the leg. Standing steadily on one leg, make the three joints of the ilium, knee and ankle of the other leg do such actions as swinging, kicking, shaking and rotating in six directions, enabling the three joints to move freely. It might be exercised selectively with reference to the sections on the practice of methods. To strengthen the balance control function of the legs, one may practice the method of kicking the Archilles tendons during walking, that is, while walking slowly, one leg falls to the ground and stands firmly, then the other leg rises, and before it advances it kicks the heel and shank of the other leg with the back of the foot. (Fig. 3-73)

[Functions]

Locally it may prevent and treat disorders such as leg pain, leg edema, spasms, numbness, paralysis, atrophy and lassitude of lower extremities, cold and pain of joints, arthroncus of knee, edema of foot and shank, angitis, phlebitis and heel pain. Distantly it benefits the waist, reinforces the kidney, regulates the stomach and strengthens the spleen. It has the effects of expelling cold and wind, promoting the flow of blood, relieving pain, clearing and activating the meridians and collaterals, and lubricating the joints.

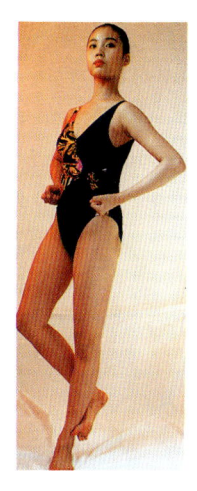

Fig. 3-73 Kicking

12. The Method to Warm Yongquan and Nourish *Yin*

This is a method to nip and pinch the toes and push and rub the sole, especially the location of the acupoint Yongquan. The foot is the part of the body that bears the greatest weight, as well as the lowest extremity, and is the place to where the morbid *qi* of the body falls. The toes are places where the three *Yin* and three *Yang* meridians of the foot converge, and the acupoint Yongquan is the starting point of the Kidney Meridian of Foot-*Shaoyin*. According to traditional Chinese medicine, the various regions of the sole are closely related to the viscera of the body, similar to the phenomenon that there are reflection points on the auricle regularly corresponding to the parts of the body. This theory has been proved by the relevant studies of modern medicine. Local health massage is not only effective on the foot region, but may also produce certain regulating, preventive and treatment effects on the whole body, serving the purposes of sending up the lucid *Yang*, nourishing kidney-*yin* and inducing fire of deficiency type.

[Procedures of Performance]

A. Nipping and pinching the toes. Assume the sitting position. Bend one or both legs into the shape of the number "4" and place it on the other leg, as required by the convenience of the performance. Apply the handwork of nipping with the thumb. First nip the tips of the toes, from the big toe to the little toe in due order. Then along the toenail groove and the dorsoventral boundary of the foot nip around the nail for a circle, until there appear redness and pain. Then apply the handwork of pinching, six times for each toe. This may also be coordinated by pulling and stretching the toes. For this action, refer to the toe-pulling method.

B. Pushing and rubbing the sole. Bend one

leg into the shape of the number "4" and place it on the other leg, or bend the leg into a kneeling position with the sole facing upward; concentrate the mind on the location of the acupoint Yongquan. Use the thumb or the base of palm of one hand to push and rub vertically from the central of the sole to the tips of the toes. One may also push and rub horizontally, or first knead and then push and rub, and use the other hand to nip and knead the acupoint Sanyinjiao. Pay attention to the speed and force. Push and rub until there appears warmness. Or one may assume the supine position, put the soles together and rub them against each other repeatedly, until there appears warmness. This method may also exercise the ilium and knee regions at the same time. The above actions are usually done before sleep after washing the feet. (Fig. 3-74)

[Functions]

Locally it may prevent and treat numbness and cold of foot, beriberi, foot edema, rhagadia, chilblain, angitis, peripheral neuritis. Generally it may prevent and treat disorders such as dizziness, heart palpitation headache, faint, epilepsy, loss of voice, nasal obstruction, acne, black eyelids, oneirogmus, insomnia, hypertension, laryngopharyngitis.

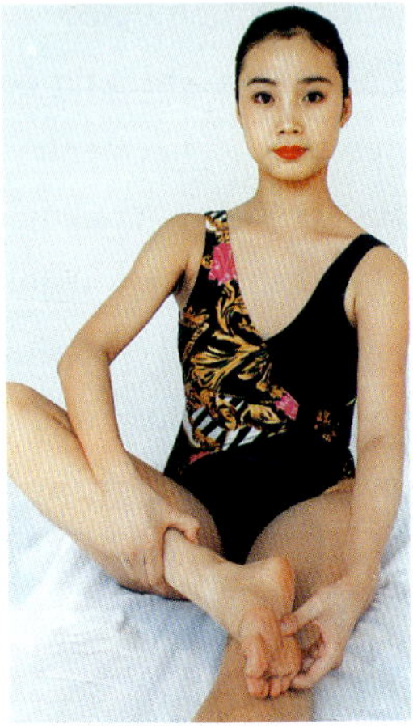

It has the effects of nourishing *yin* to reduce pathogenic fire, refreshing the mind, clearing obstruction and leading morbid *qi* to flow down. This method is easy, but has great functions.

Fig. 3-74 Pushing and rubbing Yongquan, and nipping and kneading Sanyinjiao.

13. The Method to Activate the Abdomen and Press Dantian

The abdomen is the habitat for the liver, spleen and kidney and is connencted with the stomach, intestines and gall bladder. The Conception Vessel runs across it, the *Chong* Vessel starts from it and the Belt Vessel runs around it. It is dominated by the three *yin* meridians of the foot and the meridians of Foot-*Yangming*. It is the base of energy transformation, being the origin of congenital energy and the source of acquired energy. The areas of the abdomen are hard to define clearly. Customarily, the area around the acupoint Zhongwan is referred to as the upper abdomen; the area around the acupoint Shenque, namely the umbilicus, is referred to as the middle abdomen, or the umbilical abdomen; the two sides under the ribs are referred to as the minor abdomen; and the area below the umbilicus is the lower abdomen, and the location around the acupoints Qihai and Guanyuan is referred to as Dantian. The abdomen is of *yin* nature and likes warmth and unobstructedness. When performing this method, relax the abdomen and coordinate with rhythmical respiration. Never hold breath or bulge the abdomen.

[Procedures of Performance]

A. Kneading and rubbing the abdomen. Assume the sitting or supine position. Use one hand, or two hands alternatively, to knead and rub the abdomen circularly, with the umbilicus (Shenque) as the center. Take the right hand as an example: put the palm on the upper abdomen, then from the left minor abdomen to the lower part of the lower abdomen, then up to the right minor abdomen and to the upper abdomen, knead and rub down to the middle abdomen, and point the center of the palm at Shenque. This forms one complete performance. The left hand performs in the opposite direction. Each hand does ten-odd times.

This exercise can be done according to need. For example, for fullness in chest and abdomen, it can be coordinated by pushing and rubbing the chest, pushing and rubbing from the chest or the upper abdomen through the middle abdomen to the lower abdomen. For the sinking of *qi* of the middle energizer or gastroptosis, one should push, rub and knead from the lower abdomen upward. (Fig. 3-75)

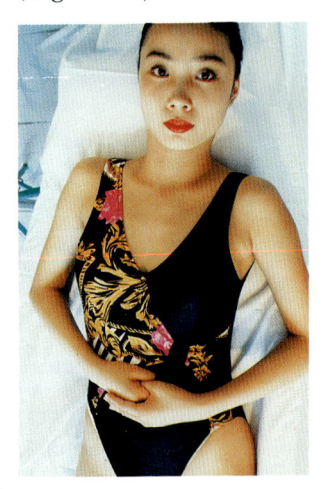

Fig. 3-75 Rubbing the abdomen.

B. Punching Shenque. Lie supine. Use the middle finger to punch the location of Shenque, until the abdomen feels distended, numb, trembling and vibrating. Or select the important acupoints on the abdomen to punch according to actual needs, such as Zhongwan, Zhangmen, Tianshu, Qihai and

Guanyuan. (Fig. 3-76)

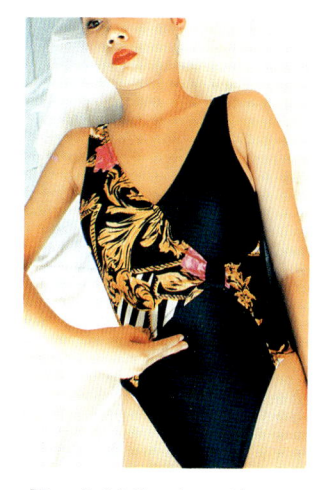

Fig. 3-76 Punching Shenque.

C. Pinching and lifting the abdominal skin. Use the thumbs and the index and middle fingers of both hands to pinch and lift the abdominal skin successively from under dovetail along the Conception Vessel directly to the lower abdomen; coordinate this exercise with vibrating actions. One may also perform from the downside to the upside. Repeat three times. (Fig. 3-77)

D. Overlap the palms and press Dantian. Lying quietly in bed before sleep, or standing in a quiet place in the morning, relax the body, tranquilize the mind, and regulate respiration. Over-

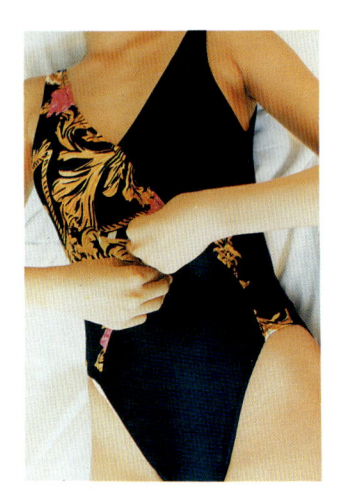

Fig. 3-77 Pinching and lifting the abdominal skin.

lap the two palms with the right hand over the left hand and the acupoints Laogong, put them on the lower abdomen, point Laogong at the acupoint Qi-hai; using the wrist to drive the palm, from the big thenar eminence to the small eminence and back to the big thenar eminence make a circular pressing motion for thirty-six circles. Then press thirty-six circles in the opposite direction, until the lower abdomen feel warm and distended. A-long with the performance, concentrate the mind on this region. Regulate the mind, and coordinate with the action of tightening the anus. When the above actions are finished, it will be better to coordinate them with bulging and rinsing the mouth to produce a mouthful of saliva, swallow it in three times and think of sending it to the lower abdomen. This action may also be exercised separately. Long-term exercise of it may refresh the spirit, strengthen health, reinforce the basis, prolong life and beautify oneself. (Fig. 3-78)

〔Functions〕

It may prevent and treat disorders such as fullness in the stomach, abdominal pain, diarrhea, constipation, dyspepsia, gastroptosis, gastric and duodenal bulbar ulcers, gastrointestinal neurosis, chronic colitis, chronic hepatitis, hemorrhoid complicated by anal fistula or prolapse of rectum, stranguria, enuresis, urinary incontinence, uroschesis, seminal emission, spermatorrhea, impotence, prospermia, dysmenorrhea, irregular menstruation and leukorrhea with reddish discharge. It has the effects of strengthening the spleen and stomach, soothing the liver and regulating the circulation of *qi*, reg-

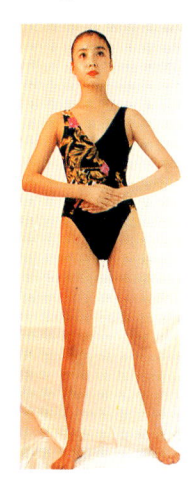

Fig. 3-78 Pressing Dantian with overlapped palms.

ulating the *Chong* and the Conception Vessels, tonifying the kidney-*qi*, regulating the uterus, lessening dampness, lowering the adverse flow of *qi*, regulating *qi* and blood, warming *yang* and treating prostration syndrome, and replenishing vital essence and reinforcing primordial *qi*. This method has fine therapeutic effects on many disorders affecting beauty, and has miraculous effects for the prevention of diseases and the care of health in the course of time.

14. The Method to Consolidate Primordial *Qi* and Strengthen *Yang*

This is a health method of self massage mainly to stimulate the external genital organs (the perineum, scrotum and penis). The external organs are pathways of the liver meridian and the Conception and the Governor Vessels. They are organs of congenital essence and have the functions of reproduction and heredity. The perineum is the place where the Conception and the Governor Vessels converge, the scrotum is the source which generates semen, and the penis is the urogenital organ. Exercise of this method may consolidate primordial *qi*, strengthen the essence, replenish vital essence and blood and invigorate the kidney-*yang*. This method mostly applies to middle-aged and old people and those suffering from decline of sexual function. Normally unmarried young people are advised not to exercise this method. After exercise of this method there may appear high sexual desire, at this time sexual activity should be moderately controlled. Never apply this method to indulge in intemperate sexual life and impair health. Exercise of this method should be coordinated by the exercise of some static nourishing methods to produce higher effects. Usually it may be exercised in combination with the Method to Activate the Abdomen and Press Dantian. Continual exercise of this method is one of the remedies for preservation of essence, longevity and good health.

[Procedures of Performance]

A. Pressing and kneading the perineum. Expose the external genital organs, sit upright, tranquilize the mind, breathe quietly, and relax the body. Press the left hand on the Dantian region, and use the middle finger of the right hand to knead the perineum, for thirty-six times clockwise and counterclockwise respectively, until there appear warmness and slight numbness. Note not to apply too much force or too quick a speed. Remember to concentrate the mind and knead the perineum lightly and slowly. It will be better to coordinate with the action of lifting the anus for the prevention and treatment of anal and intestinal disorders. For females the actions are the same as above.

B. Propping the scrotum. Use the middle finger to flick and press the base of the scrotum (testicles) near the perineum. After that, prop and rub the testicles and the penis upward to nestle it close against the lower abdomen. Do it with each hand alternatively, for one hundred-odd times, until there appear sensations of distention, soreness and warmness. The force and speed may be increased gradually.

For females, use the middle finger to press and knead the acupoints Guanyuan, Zhongji and Qugu counterclockwise, for 60 to 90 times, with such force as to produce slight soreness and distention. Do not press and knead too heavily.

C. Pinching and scrubbing the external genitals. Hold the testicles with both hands, the thumb and index finger forcefully pinch and knead the two testicles with such force as to produce slight tolerable soreness and pain. Do not exert too much force. Then pinch the penis and twist it outward from its base, until there appear distention and pain and the penis slightly erects. Finally hold the testicles and the penis between the two palms and the small thenar eminences exert force against each other to scrub and move from the inside to the outside and from the downside to the upside. Determine the times of action according to one's own physical conditions.

For females, mainly rub the vulva about 30 times.

Unmarried young men and women are advised not to exercise this method lest there appear deviations.

Besides the above, there are other methods such as beating with the palm, beating with a stick, grasping and stroking, and hanging weights. They are not introduced here.

[Functions]

It can prevent and treat disorders such as impotence, prospermia, spermatorrhea, spontaneous emission, prostitis, decline of sexual function, lumbago due to the kidney deficiency, coldness of abdomen and loose stool, hemorrhoid complicated by anal fistrla or prolapse of rectum, amnesia, insomnia, irregular menstruation, leukorrhea, obesity, pathologic leanness, black eyelids and freckles. It has the effects of tonifying the kidney, reinforcing the brain, controlling nocturnal emission, strengthening *yang*, prolonging life and building up health. This is one of the fine beautifying methods.

Part IV

Massotherapy for Common Disorders Affecting Beauty

This part introduces the massotherapy for some common disorders affecting beauty, such as facial wrinkles, roughness of skin, freckles, acne, baldness, strabismus, scars, facial paralysis, dim, sallow or pale complexion, mammary maldevelopment, atrophy of gum, obesity and pathologic leanness. Some of these disorders cannot be treated with massage alone and have to be treated in coordination with proper drugs and other therapies. Dim complexion, for example, can be caused by many factors, either mental depression, or physical weakness, or the liver and kidney deficiecy of the *yin* type, or irregular menstruation or endocrine disorder. Nevertheless, massotherapy, especially local beauty massage, does have certain effects and will complement with other therapies in coordination. However, with respect to delaying senility and keeping beauty, beauty massage can make "special contributions".

In the previous part on the methods, the prevention and treatment of disorders affecting beauty have already been introduced. In this part, the processes of performance will not be elaborated. The methods are presented in the form of prescriptions.

Facial Wrinkles

Wrinkles are a phenomenon of the aging of the skin. Generally speaking, wrinkles on the forehead appear the earliest, to be followed by laughter wrinkles and wrinkles by the corner of the eye. They are mostly due to long-term spiritual tension, excessive anxiety, disorder of the digestive function, lowering of the hormone level, disturbance in the blood circulation of the capillaries and imbalance of nutrition. They are a phenomenon of aging.

〔Beauty Prescription〕

A. Massage the whole body once.

B. Focus on doing the Method to Activate the Abdomen and Press Dantian and the Method to Consolidate Primordial *Qi* and Strengthen *Yang*.

C. Repeat the Method to Strengthen the Mind and Beautify the Face three to five times.

D. Do one treatment of face membrane of self-prepared egg white and honey every three days.

[Points of Attention]

A. Keep a happy mood, have enough sleep and increase nutrition.

B. Properly coordinate massage with taking vitamins needed by one's body and traditional Chineae drugs strengthening the brain, tonifying the kidney, promoting blood circulation and removing blood stasis. Also coordinate with medicated baths.

Dim Complexion

Dim complexion is usually caused by deficiency of the liver and kidney, noncoordination between the spleen and the stomach, subnutrition and disturbance of blood circulation. The remedy is to tonify the liver and kidney, strengthen the spleen, regulate the stomach, promote blood circulation and remove blood stasis to brighten and moisten the complexion.

[Beauty Prescription]

A. Massage the whole body once.

B. Focus on doing the Method to Strengthen the Waist and Tonify the Kidney, the Method to Activate the Abdomen and Press Dantian and the

Method to Warm Yongquan and Nourish *Yin*.

C. Repeat the Method to Strengthen the Mind and Beautify the Face and the Intraoral Method for Longevity three to five times.

D. Do one time of face membrane of fruits every other day.

[Points of Attention]

A. Relax the mind, have enough rest and do moderate exercise.

B. Coordinate with drugs tonifying the liver and kidney, strengthening the brain and regulating the stomach.

Freckles (Brown Spots and Butterfly Spots)

Freckles are black or brown pigmented spots. Their occurrence is probably related to hereditary factors, mental depression, weakness of the functions of the liver and kidney, and stagnancy of *qi* and blood stasis. Butterfly spots are mostly seen in females suffering from irregular menstruation, during pregnancy and after delivery, symmetrical on the left and right and with clear outlines. Treatment should be given in accordance with the different causes, mainly to tonify the liver and kidney, regulate the circulation of *qi* and blood, improve local blood circulation and balance the level of hormone secretion, to eliminate or reduce freckles.

〔Beauty Prescription〕

A. Massage the whole body once.

B. Focus on doing the Method to Expand the Chest and Costa, the Method to Warm Yongquan and Nourish *Yin*, the Method to Warm Yongquan and Nourish *Yin* and the Intraoral Method for Longevity.

C. Repeat the Method to Beautify the Complexion and Brighten the Eyes, the Method to Induce Resuscitation and Clear Nasal Passage and the Method to Strengthen the Nind and Beautify the Face. Do each for six times every evening and morning. The performance should be slow, to be coordinated with traditional Chinese drugs such as Chinese angelica or safflower preparations to promote blood circulation and remove freckles.

〔Points of Attention〕

A. Keep a happy mood, relax the mind, and have enough sleep.

B. For ordinary brown spots, take orally some vitamin E or traditional Chinese preparations that tonify the kidney and liver, promote blood circulation and remove blood stasis.

235

Make face membranes by mixing equal amounts of tomato juice and honey, and apply one on the face in the morning and evening. For the key locations the density of the membrane may be thicker. Usually apply the membrane on the face after beauty massage is finished. Apply the membrane to the face once a week

C. For butterfly spots in females, coordinate treatment with regulating menstruation. Do not apply any drugs during pregnancy lest the fetus be affected. After delivery, focus on treating postpartum disorders and coordinate with face membranes and massage.

Acne

Acne is mostly seen on oleaginous skin. In normal people, sebum cutaneum is discharged out of the body through the pores of sebaceous glands. If the pores are obstructed affecting the discharge of the sebum, germ infection will cause local inflammation which greatly affects and impairs the beauty of the face. According to traditional Chinese medicine's differentiation of the symptoms and signs, acne can be divided into the types of dampness and heat of the liver and spleen, deficiency-fire of the lung and kidney and infection of toxic heat. The treatment should focus on eliminating dampness and heat, purging fire and removing stasis, and clearing away heat and toxins. That is, focus on regulating the spleen and kidney, reducing hormone secretion and alleviating inflammation to clean and smoothen the face.

〔Beauty Prescription〕

A. Massage the whole body once.

B. Focus on doing the Method to Expand the Chest and Costa, the Method to Warm Yongquan and Nourish *Yin* and the Method to Activate the Abdomen and Press Dantian.

C. Repeat the Method to Induce Resuscitation and Clear Nasal Passage and the Method to Strengthen the Mind and Beautify the Face. Do each for six times in the morning and evening respectively. For coordination, take proper acne ointments at the media, or smear one's own saliva.

D. Do a face membrane of lemon or citrus juice once a day, or smear cucumber juice on the face.

〔Points of Attention〕

A. Avoid restlessness, have enough sleep and pay attention to exercise.

B. Do not take pungent, fishy, muttony or

fatty food. Refrain from smoking and drinking. Eat fruits and vegetables frequently.

C. Do not abuse so-called beautifying and nourishing cosmetics.

D. For coordination, take traditional Chinese drugs and preparations removing damp-heat from the liver and the gallbladder, alleviating inflammation and purging fire, promoting blood circulation and removing blood stasis, as well as Western vitamins C and B.

Rough Skin

Rough skin occurs easily in dry skin. With sunburn it will change color and peel off, and in cold weather it will chap and drop furfurs. Rough skin is mostly caused by deficiency of qi and blood, stagnancy of qi and blood stasis, dysfunction of the viscera and nutritious substances' incapability of moistening the skin.

[Beauty Prescription]

A. Massage the whole body once.

B. Focus on doing the Method to Strengthen the Waist and Tonify the Kidney, the Method to Activate the Abdomen and Press Dantian, the Method to Consolidate Primordial Qi and

Strengthen *Yang* and the Method to warm Yongquan and Nourish *Yin*.

C. Repeat the Method to Beautify the Face and Relax the Neck and the Method to Strengthen the Mind and Beautify the Face three times every moring and evening.

D. Do one treatment of face membrane of milk powder, yolk and honey every other day.

[Points of Attention]

A. Have enough sleep, exercise moderately and increase nutrition.

B. Reduce the use of alkaline soaps. Pay attention to avoiding cold, hotness, wind and sunburn.

Pale Complexion

Fair skin demonstrates health and beauty, and pale and dim complexion indicates morbidity. Pale complexion is mostly seen in cases of malnutrition, anemia and physical weakness. At the same time of increasing nutrition and treating in time, it will be beneficial to do beauty massage frequently.

[Beauty Prescription]

A. Massage the whole body three times each day.

B. Focus on doing the Method to Activate the Abdomen and Press Dantian, the Method to Consolidate Primordial *Qi* and Strengthen *Yang*, the Intraoral Method for Longevity and the Method to Strengthen the Mind and Beautify the Face.

C. Do one treatment of face membrane of yolk, honey and glycerine every other day.

[Points of Attention]

A. Keep a happy mood, increase nutrition and exercise properly.

B. Treat the underlying disorders in accordance with the need.

Facial Paralysis

Facial paralysis is mostly caused by facial exposure to cold wind or excessive anger. For facial paralysis caused by cerebrovascular diseases, the stress should be laid on treating the underlying diseases. Treatment of general facial paralysis with massage aims at clearing and activating meridians, promoting blood circulation and removing blood stasis.

[Beauty Prescription]

A. Massage the whole body once in the morning and evening respectively.

B. Focus on doing the Method to Expand the Chest and Costa, the Method to Beautify the Complexion and Brighten the Eyes, the Method to Induce Resuscitation and Clear Nasal Passage, the Method to Strengthen the Mind and Beautify the Face and the Method to Warm Yongquan and Nourish *Yin*.

C. Make a face membrane of 10 grams of scorpion, 10 grams of batryticated silkworm and 10 grams of giant typhonium tuber all ground into powder. Do one treatment of face membrane once a day, for 7 days successively.

〔Points of Attention〕

A. Keep a happy mood and have enough sleep.

B. Avoid being blown by cold wind and washing the face with cold water.

Gingival Atrophy

Gingival atrophy is mainly due to trauma or inflammation, exposing the roots of teeth partially or entirely, and is liable to cause odontoseisis and odontoptosis. It is one of the factors causing saprodontia and odontonecrosis, directly affecting food intake and digestion, making beauty all the less present. It is usually caused by insalubrity of the oral cavity. Massage is an effective method to prevent and treat this disease.

〔Beauty Prescription〕

A. Do the Method to Beautify the Face and Relax the Neck three times a day, and lay stress on doing the section of knocking the teeth in the Intraoral Method for Longevity.

B. For coordination, do the Method to Strengthen the Mind and Beautify the Face and the Method to Nourish Intelligence and Improve Hearing.

〔Points of Attention〕

Keep a stable mood, pay attention to the diet and avoid hard, cold, hot and sour foods.

Scars

Scars are projections caused by hyperplasia or lumps left on the surface of the body by trauma, operation and inflammation when they are healed. At exposed parts scars will affect beauty, and at the joints scars will impede normal functioning. Longterm persevering local massage may soften scars, reduce the teneseness of the skin, beautify the skin and ease the movement of the joints.

〔Beauty Prescription〕

Employ the finger-pressing handwork to press around the scar gradually from light to heavy. Then employ the handwork of kneading to the scar repeatedly until there appear redness and a painful sensation. After that, employ the handwork of pinching to pinch the scar ten-odd times. Finally employ the handwork of stroking or rubbing. One may properly coordinate with the application of Chinese angelica or safflower preparations that promote blood circulation as the media.

[Points of Attention]

Do not injure the skin. Frequently apply a hot towel over the scar to strengthen its ability to dissolve lumps.

Mammary Maldevelopment

In females, the breasts play a decisive role in the beauty of the chest. Mammary maldevelopment, such as hypermastia, level or lean and small breasts and crater nipples, affects the special curvilinear beauty of females.

[Beauty Prescription]

A. Massage the whole body once.

B. Focus on doing the Method to Strengthen the Waist and Tonify the Kidney, the Method to

Consolidate Primordial *Qi* and Strengthen *Yang*.

C. Repeat the section of plumping the breasts in the Method to Expand the Chest and Costa, twice a day.

〔Points of Attention〕

A. Foster a fine spiritual state, pay attention to nutrition, have enough sleep, and do chest-expanding exercises more.

B. Do not bind the chest too tightly, except in the case of hypermastia.

C. Frequently take some traditional Chinese drugs and Western vitamins that can increase hormone secretion.

Obesity

Obesity not only affects the beauty of the body but can also incur many diseases. For morbid obesity, focus on treating the primary disease. for simple obesity, focus on reducing the accumulation of subcutaneous fat and quickening the metabolism and absorption of fat.

〔Beauty Prescription〕

A. Massage the whole body once.

B. Focus on doing the Method to Strengthen the Waist and Tonify the Kidney and the Method to Expand the Chest and Costa.

C. Repeat the Method to Activate the Abdomen and Press Dantian and the Method to Beautify the Face and Relax the Neck, twice a day.

[Points of Attention]

A. Eat less, exercise more and sleep less.

B. For coordination, take effective weight-loss preparations.

C. Frequently have hot medicated baths; it is better to apply massage after the baths.

Pathologic Leanness

Excessive leanness demonstrates too little subcutaneous fat, showing depressed eye, drawn cheeks, wrinkles all over the face, level chest and hips and the disappearance of the curves of the body. Its causes are mostly related to heredity, endocrine disturbance and chronic consumptive diseases. Traditional Chinese medicine mostly regards deficiency of *qi* and blood, weakness of the spleen and the kidney, the liver and the kidney deficiency of the *yin* type and hyperactivity of *yang* due to *yin* deficiency as its pathogenic factors. Massage focuses on regulating the whole body and has double regulating effects of excitement and inhibition on the digestive system, the endocrinous system, neurohumor metabolism and glycometabolism. But the stress is laid on promoting digestion, strengthening absorption and regulating *yin* and *yang*.

[Beauty Prescription]

A. Massage the whole body twice a day.

B. Repeat the Method to Activate the Abdomen and Press Dantian, the Method to Consolidate Primordial *Qi* and Strengthen *Yang* and the Method to Strengthen the Mind and Beautify the Face.

[Points of Attention]

A. Keep a happy mood and have enough sleep.

B. Increase nutrition, especially high-protein, high-fat, high-carbohydrate foods (unless you are diabetic) and foods containing many kinds of vitamins. The basis is the diet of flavor plus nutrition.

C. Take corresponging medicines in consideration of the pathogenic factors.

Disorders affecting beauty are more than the above-mentioned twelve kinds. Other disorders such as myopia, hyperopia, strabismus, trichiasis, black eyelids, brandy nose, dorsal spots, roughness and wrinkles of fingers and flaccidity of the skin of the neck and the nape have been discussed in the part of the book on methods.

Repair the house before it rains. Take preventive measures and practise perseveringly; miraculous effects will then be achieved, ——and that is the very aim of this book!

中国美容按摩术

卞春强　陶瑜　著

荆强　马千里　摄影

胡兆云　译

哈罗德·师文德　校译

*

中国山东友谊出版社出版
(中国山东济南胜利大街39号)
中国山东新华印刷厂德州厂印刷
中国国际图书贸易总公司发行
(中国北京车公庄西路35号)
北京邮政信箱第399号　邮政编码100044
英文版
1996年4月第1版　1996年4月第1次印刷
ISBN7—80551—828—9/R·12
07600
14—E—2939P